The Complete Type 2 Diabetes Cookbook for Beginners

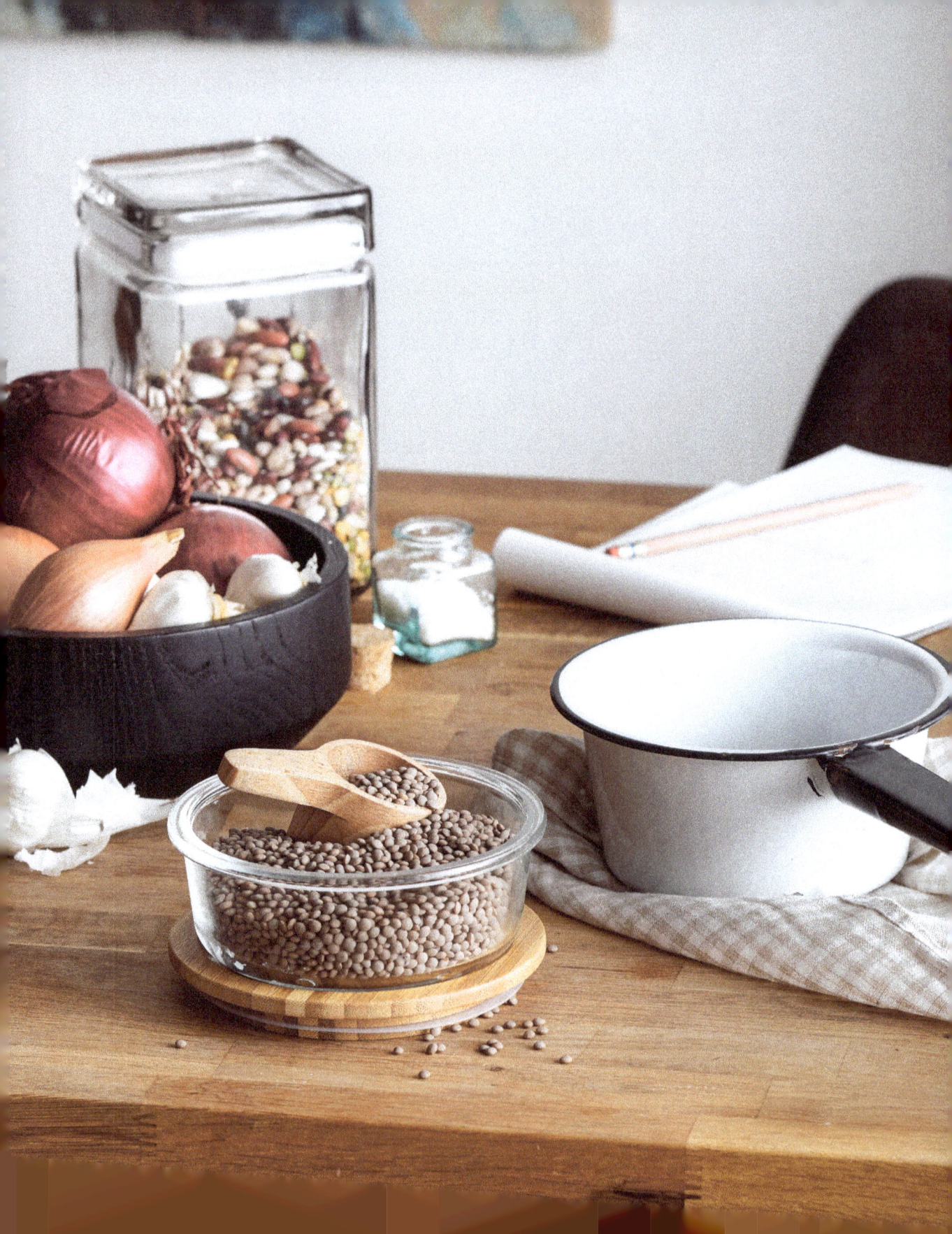

2025

THE COMPLETE
TYPE 2
DIABETES
COOKBOOK
FOR BEGINNERS

150 Easy and Heart-Healthy Recipes

Edited by
Ariel Warren, RDN, CD, CDCES

callisto
publishing
an imprint of Sourcebooks

Art Director: Darren Samuel
Art Producer: Sue Bischofberger
Editor: Georgia Freedman
Production Editor: Matthew Burnett
Production Manager: Riley Hoffman

Originally published as *Complete Type 2 Diabetes Cookbook: 150 Healthy Recipes to Manage Diabetes* in 2022 in the United States of America by Callisto Publishing, an imprint of Callisto Publishing LLC.

Published by Callisto Publishing LLC C/O Sourcebooks LLC
P.O. Box 4410, Naperville, Illinois 60567-4410
(630) 961-3900
callistopublishing.com

Printed and bound in the United States of America

I would like to dedicate this recipe book to all my friends living with diabetes. Also, to my wonderful and supportive husband and beautiful children.

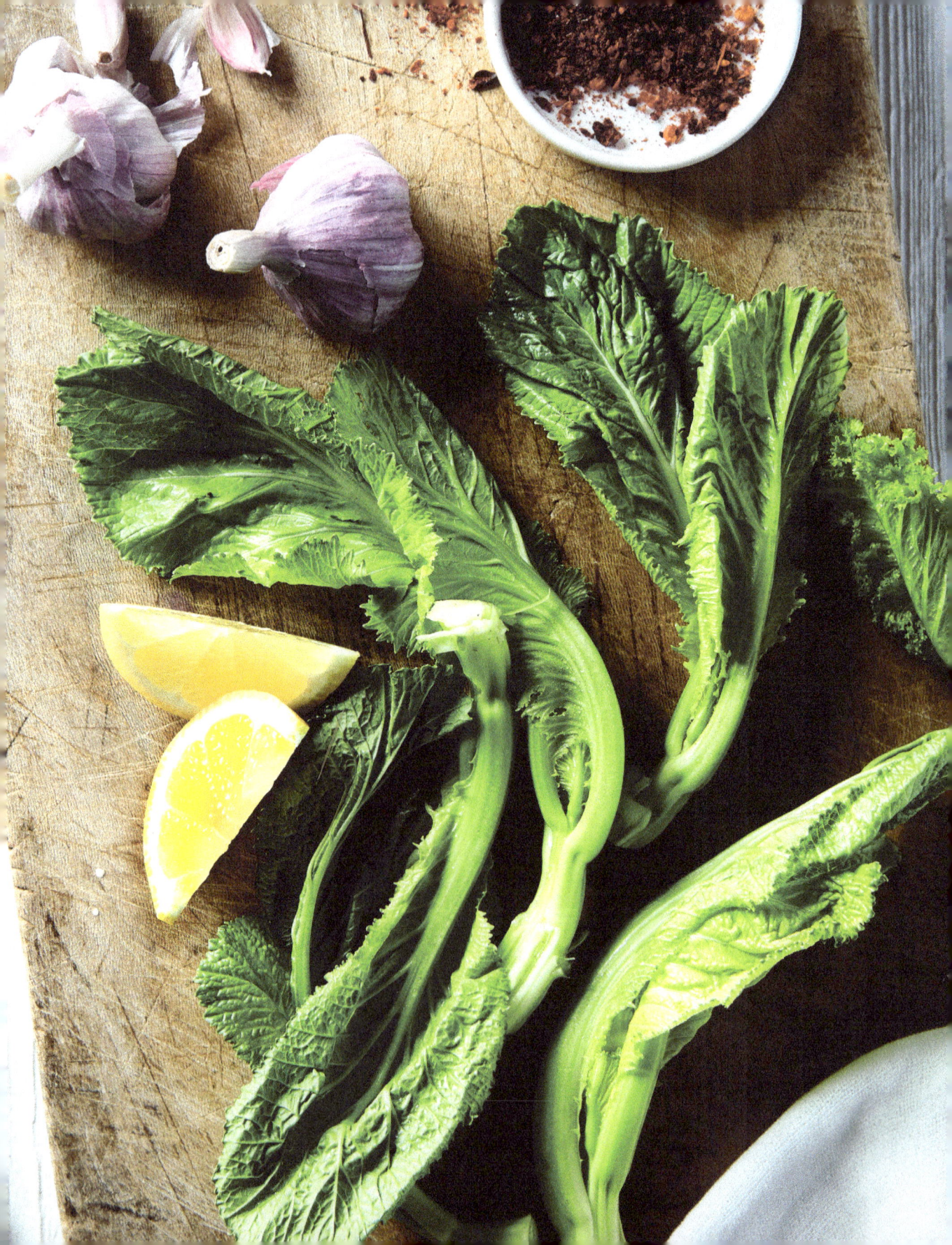

Contents

Introduction

Hello, reader! I am excited you found this diabetes-friendly cookbook. It is packed with 150 recipes to help you reach your blood sugar and health goals. Every recipe was created with you in mind. Not only do these recipes use an assortment of whole-food ingredients but they are packed with the nutrients and fiber essential for diabetes management. Each recipe also includes handy tips so you can adapt it to suit your palate.

Let me introduce myself. My name is Ariel Warren. I have had diabetes since 1995. At the age of four, I was diagnosed when we didn't have the current evidence-based research that shows how powerfully food and lifestyle habits impact blood sugar and overall quality of life. At a young age, I felt how food impacted my diabetes control and my energy. This recognition was my primary motivation for pursuing a career as a registered dietitian nutritionist (RDN) and a certified diabetes care and education specialist (CDCES). As a healthcare provider, I work with people with diabetes and for years witnessed the direct and powerful effects of food and physical activity on blood sugar levels and overall well-being.

As a dietitian and someone with diabetes, I understand that healthy eating does *not* mean we should restrict all foods not categorized as highly nutritious. A foundational part of eating healthy is cultivating a healthy *relationship* with food. Make fruits, vegetables, whole grains, and lean protein the basis of your diet, but give yourself permission to enjoy a dessert or special treat. Just make sure your medication is adjusted accordingly. I realize this is easier said than done if you have spent years dieting and restricting. Developing a healthy relationship with food takes time and support. Be kind to yourself. I strongly feel that the best way of eating when you have diabetes is to consume healthier versions of the food you already enjoy. It is much easier to form sustainable, healthy habits by sticking to foods you like.

The best way to eat for most people with diabetes is balanced meals using the diabetes plate method: a meal of 50 percent non-starchy vegetables, 25 percent starch or grains, and 25 percent protein. These meals use naturally filling and nutritious foods, and they provide better blood sugar control and energy levels. That said, everyone managing their diabetes will have to find the best carbohydrate amount for their goals.

Carbohydrates are a very hot topic in the world of diabetes. Many people do not fully understand that when diabetes is properly managed with exercise, medication, and/or insulin, you can still safely eat carbohydrates and have great blood sugar control. Personally, I love carbohydrates. Yes, I know they need to be balanced with fiber, protein, and healthy fats, but carbohydrates are the primary fuel source to produce energy for your body and brain. Also, the fiber in many carbohydrates aids in digestion, helps you feel full, reduces cholesterol levels, and has been found to reduce many types of cancer. If you do better with lower carbs, you can bulk up on the non-starchy foods and protein sources found in recipes throughout this book and use the carbohydrate portion as more of a garnish.

No matter where you're coming from—whether you're newly diagnosed or a long-time veteran of diabetes—this book will provide you with choices that are delicious, well-balanced, and allow for improved blood sugar control and health.

This book is meant to provide various kinds of healthy meals to suit a wide variety of people. If you have specific guidelines that work best for you, you will find recipes that fit your individualized needs. You will find a wide range of recipes, from breakfast smoothies to sandwiches, from vegan meals to meaty mains. Altogether, this collection contains everything you need to make super satisfying meals and the information to ensure you're well equipped to improve your diabetes care.

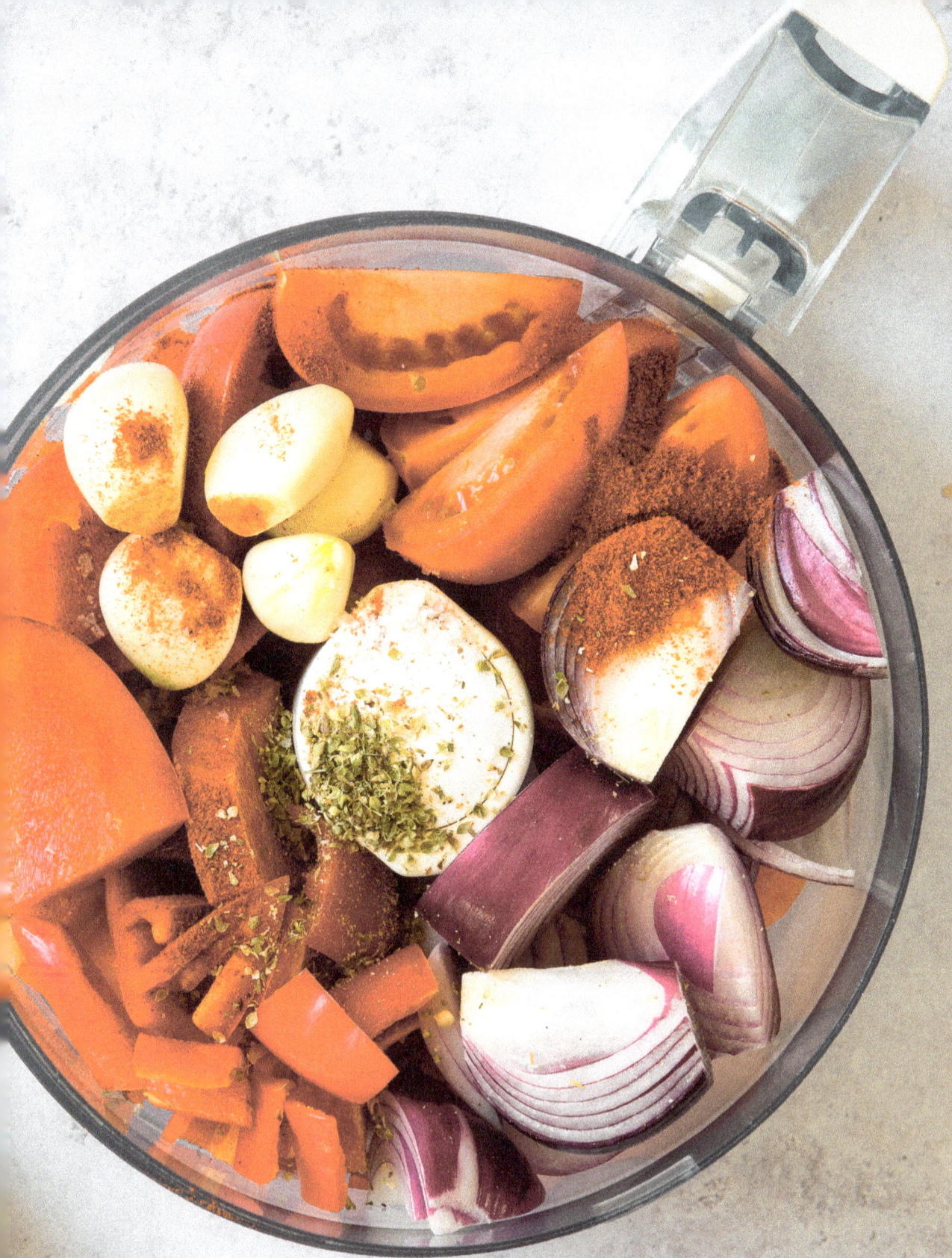

1

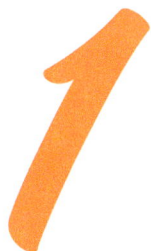

THE COMPLETE DIABETES DIET AND LIFESTYLE

Nutrition and physical activity are crucial components of living a healthy life, with or without diabetes. While healthy eating should always be a priority, when you have diabetes, the impact from healthy foods and regular exercise will be more immediate. As someone who has lived with diabetes for many years, I realized early on that I felt better overall, my mood and energy levels were higher, and my blood sugar was more stable when I ate balanced and nutritious foods and exercised. After several years of education and paying attention to how direct this impact is, I have chosen to see diabetes as a positive motivator.

WHAT DOES IT MEAN TO HAVE TYPE 2 DIABETES?

According to the Centers for Disease Control and Prevention (CDC), the National Diabetes Statistics Report in 2020 estimated that about 34.2 million people have diabetes (10.5 percent of Americans). There are about 26.9 million people (26.8 million adults) diagnosed, and about 7.3 million who have diabetes but are undiagnosed.

There are roughly 88 million people aged 18 years or older (34.5 percent of the adult US population) with prediabetes, including about 24.2 million people aged 65 or older (see Prediabetes on page 5 for more information). While most estimates of diabetes in this report do not differentiate between type 1 diabetes (T1D) and type 2 diabetes (T2D), T2D accounts for 90 to 95 percent of all diabetes cases. Therefore, most of the people represented in the CDC Statistics Report's data have T2D.

My point is there are many people with diabetes, especially T2D. This information can be helpful, because it allows us to increase understanding and know we are not alone as we navigate new dietary advice and learn how to live a healthy and full life with diabetes. Being diagnosed with diabetes can be confusing, and, even if you've managed T2D for a while, the extent of information available is difficult to wade through and remember. So, I've broken down the information in a clear, easy-to-understand way.

Diabetes

Usually, when someone without diabetes eats, food is broken down into glucose (sugar) so the body can use it for energy. The body produces the hormone insulin in the beta cells in the pancreas, and insulin transports the glucose from the food into the cells so it can be used for energy. When someone has diabetes—due to either a lack of insulin (T1D) or insulin resistance (T2D)—the glucose from food cannot be properly transported into the body's cells, so the sugar (glucose) remains in the blood creating a high blood sugar level that can cause complications for the body and brain.

Diabetes has many subclassifications—T1D and T2D are the two main subtypes—and each has a different pathophysiology, presentation, and management solution. But all subtypes can cause high blood sugar and become life-threatening if left untreated.

T1D is an autoimmune condition where the body attacks the beta cells of the pancreas so it only produces very little insulin or none. This causes the person to become insulin-dependent. T2D occurs when insufficient insulin is released into the bloodstream or the insulin cannot be used properly. Someone with T2D may actually produce higher amounts of insulin compared to someone without T2D. The body senses the high blood sugar levels and signals the pancreas to produce more and more insulin. Unfortunately, the body is unable to use the insulin, due to the decreased ability of the cells to absorb and use the glucose for energy. Also, T2D is a progressive condition, so someone with T2D may require increased amounts of exogenous insulin to compensate over time.

Experiencing slight fluctuations in blood sugar levels in response to food is completely normal, even for people without diabetes. Blood sugar between 60 to 140 mg/dL (milligrams per deciliter) is considered healthy for everyone. Someone's blood sugar can have brief excursions outside this range and still be considered normal. However, blood sugar above 140 mg/dL is hyperglycemia (high blood sugar). If you don't add insulin, the organs cannot use the extra glucose, so it builds up. If T1D is untreated, blood glucose levels can rise to over 500 mg/dL. However, blood sugar this elevated is uncommon for people with T2D. Conversely, blood sugar below 60 mg/dL is considered low, which can also be dangerous. Just adding insulin isn't the only answer to diabetes treatment. Managing diabetes well is a balancing act. Adequately dosing and timing medication along with exercising and eating balanced meals containing good sources of protein, healthy fats, and complex carbohydrates with fiber can help people with either type of diabetes maintain healthy blood sugar control.

People with T2D may have high blood sugar for many years before it causes any noticeable physical symptoms. When high blood sugar does present, it can cause extreme thirst, tiredness, frequent urination, dizziness, and nausea in the short term. Long-term effects include damage to the large and small blood vessels, which increases the chances of heart attack, stroke, and problems with the brain, kidneys, eyes, feet, and nerves.

People with T2D typically only get low blood sugar when using insulin (or blood-sugar-lowering medications) to reduce high blood sugar and take a dose too large for their needs. Unexpected exercise, not eating enough food, or drinking too much alcohol can cause someone to need less insulin than intended, which drops the blood sugar below normal. Signs of low blood sugar include headaches, confusion, racing pulse, cold sweats, extreme hunger, shaking, or feeling weak, tired, restless, and/or anxious. The intensity of these symptoms depends on many factors, including how fast and by how much the blood sugar is dropping, what the person's normal blood sugar range is, and how long the person has had low blood sugar. Mild low blood sugar is uncomfortable but doesn't usually lead to serious consequences. However, severely low blood sugar can cause loss of consciousness and seizures, which can become life-threatening if left untreated.

Yes, diabetes can be a little scary, but by choosing a healthy lifestyle and the right medical team and treatment, you can delay or prevent complications. Even if you haven't been great with your care in the past, you can still make changes now. Part of that process is being proactive with screenings to detect any diabetes-related health problems early. Another is keeping your waistline, blood pressure, blood glucose levels, hemoglobin A1c (see page 6), and cholesterol levels within recommended ranges. Using healthy recipes (like the ones in this book) is an excellent way to jump-start these changes.

Prediabetes

Prediabetes is when your blood sugar is higher than normal but not high enough for a doctor to diagnose you with T2D. If left untreated, prediabetes can develop into T2D, so it is essential to make lifestyle changes and work with your medical team quickly when you're diagnosed.

As a registered dietitian nutritionist and a diabetes educator, the first recommendation I give for prediabetes is lifestyle changes. Think of a prediabetes diagnosis as your signal to act by changing eating and exercise habits so you can prevent developing T2D. According to the CDC, losing 5 to 7 percent of your body weight (just 10 to 14 pounds for someone weighing 200 pounds) will significantly lower your chances of developing T2D. Eating a balanced, nutrient-dense diet keeps you at a calorie deficit (you burn more energy than you consume), and this, along with regular activity, can help you achieve the weight loss necessary to reduce your T2D risk. Sustainable weight loss is achieved by behavior changes, not restriction. So, by eating a healthier diet and developing a positive relationship with food, you will be much better equipped for a transformation that sticks.

What do I mean by regular exercise? Generally, this means getting about 150 minutes of activity—brisk walking, bike riding, swimming, weight training, or even shoveling snow—each week, which is about 30 minutes a day, five days a week. If 30 minutes at a time is difficult, you can break it up! Sneak in 15 minutes before your day starts and the other 15 around lunch or after dinner. Over time, these small changes will have a significant impact.

All about Blood Sugar Levels

There are several ways to diagnose diabetes. While testing for blood sugar with a blood test meter is the primary way, another common method is the A1c test—also known as the hemoglobin A1c or HbA1c test. This test measures the average blood sugar levels over two to three months: the higher the percentage, the higher your average blood sugar has been during this time period. A doctor will often use this at diagnosis and check it every three to six months to help you and your healthcare team monitor how well your current treatment plan is working.

If you do not present with high blood sugar symptoms at diagnosis but the HbA1c test or another blood sugar test shows high blood sugar, repeat the test on a different day, using the HbA1c test or other diabetes blood meter test to confirm the diagnosis. You can test with a home blood glucose meter to check yourself, but testing with a meter should be performed in a healthcare setting for an official diagnosis.

Blood Sugar Ranges for Normal, Prediabetes, and Diabetes

	Blood Sugar Range [A1c Range]
NORMAL	Less than 5.7 percent
PREDIABETIC	5.7 to 6.4 percent
DIABETIC	6.5 percent or higher

Does Diabetes Ever Go Away?

When someone is diagnosed with T2D, it never completely goes away. There isn't a cure. Remission is the more accurate term to describe someone who reverts to normal blood sugar levels without medication. The term "remission" is more appropriate because blood sugar levels constantly change, minute by minute, due to eating, sleeping, exercise, stress, sickness, hormones, medication, weight, and many other factors.

Weight is an important consideration because gaining it, particularly abdominal fat around the waistline, contributes to insulin resistance and, thus, type 2 diabetes. There are two different types of fat: subcutaneous fat (just under the skin) and visceral fat (also called abdominal fat) which wraps around the abdominal organs deep inside the body. An article published in the BMC Endocrine Disorders in 2018 stated that carrying a high amount of visceral fat can lead to glucose intolerance because visceral fat secretes a protein called retinol-binding protein 4 (RBP4) which has been linked to obesity and shown to increase insulin resistance.

The higher the visceral fat, the higher the insulin resistance, the greater the chances of developing type 2 diabetes, and the more medication and/or insulin is often required to control blood sugar levels. However, if someone loses weight, especially visceral fat, it improves their body's insulin sensitivity.

When someone becomes more insulin sensitive, they require fewer medications and less insulin. By losing enough weight—especially visceral fat and in the early stages of a T2D diagnosis—you can significantly lower blood sugar levels, reduce long-term complications, and set yourself up for a much higher chance of achieving T2D remission. Moreover, if someone has only had diabetes for a short period with higher pancreatic function (the pancreas produces a more normal amount of insulin), then there is a greater chance of achieving T2D remission.

Medication

While healthy eating and exercise should be the basis of diabetes treatment, medications are also commonly used to help bring the blood sugar back to healthy ranges. It's important to closely monitor your eyes, feet, kidneys, and nerves, and to have routine blood work so that your doctor knows which medications provide the most benefit for your specific health needs and goals. There are several different groups of medications used for treating diabetes. Some even benefit multiple organs by increasing insulin sensitivity (so that less insulin is required), helping with weight loss, and protecting the heart and kidneys. However, before taking any medication, always review potential adverse side effects with your healthcare provider.

With T2D, you have many options for medications and combinations of medications. However, because T2D is a progressive disease, your body may not produce enough insulin for your needs even with your medication regimen, so insulin will likely be prescribed. You may only need insulin for a short period—during something stressful or an illness, for instance—or you may require insulin over the long term. There is absolutely nothing wrong with taking insulin. Over time, you will likely manage your diabetes with your medical team in many ways, with different medications (including possibly insulin) and in different amounts. What's important is to monitor your blood sugar and blood work, screen to prevent complications, and work with your medical team so you can find the right treatment for you.

Type 2 FAQ

Which type of diabetes do I have?

T2D is the most common type of diabetes and may present with the following symptoms: increased thirst, frequent urination, increased hunger, tingling, pain, or numbness in the arms or feet, blurred vision, slow-healing sores, and frequent infections.

T2D and T1D have very similar symptoms. However, T2D symptoms often develop more slowly, while the onset for someone with T1D develops quickly.

If you are unsure of the type of diabetes, you should get additional testing. It's possible you could have T1D (previously called juvenile diabetes), which is more commonly diagnosed in children, teens, and young adults but can develop at any age.

There is also latent autoimmune diabetes in adults (LADA), a less-common form of autoimmune diabetes that affects adults over 35 years old and has some of the same signs and symptoms as both T1D and T2D which can make a LADA diagnosis more challenging.

CONTINUED ▶

Type 2 FAQ (CONTINUED)

What tests and screening should be done now?

If you have a relatively recent T2D diagnosis, ask your doctor if you should screen for diabetes complications. If you've known about your diabetes and have been managing it for a while, make sure your screenings and tests are up to date. Common screenings look for eye problems, nerve damage, circulation problems, high cholesterol, high blood pressure, and kidney disease.

How often should I test my blood sugar?

How often you test will depend on the state of your diabetes and your treatment plan. Doctors often recommend at least a fasting blood sugar test in the morning before food or drinking anything but water for many patients. If you are on medications known to drop your blood sugar or are prescribed insulin, your doctor will likely recommend you to test multiple times a day. If you are given this recommendation, ask about a continuous glucose monitor (CGM), which continuously checks your blood sugar every few minutes through a tiny sensor inserted temporarily under your skin.

What should my blood sugar goal targets be?

According to the American Diabetes Association (ADA), the recommended blood sugar target is 80 to 130 mg/dL before meals and less than 180 mg/dL 1 to 2 hours after the start of a meal. However, your doctor may have specific blood sugar targets for you relating to your treatment, medical history, age, and other factors affecting your diabetes. So, it's always best to ask.

If starting on medication, what are the side effects?

Before starting any medication, your doctor should do an in-depth review of your medical history to see if you have any contraindications. If you do start a new medication, ask what side effects to expect and how long they typically last. If you have difficult side effects, talk to your doctor, but never stop a medication without consulting with your doctor first. Some side effects are temporary. Common side effects with T2D medications include gastrointestinal issues such as nausea, loss of appetite, upset stomach, diarrhea, or flatulence. Depending on the type of medication, you may also experience dizziness, muscle fatigue, weakness or unusual tiredness, and/or headaches. Make sure to talk to your doctor if your side effects are severe or are not going away after a few weeks.

MANAGING DIABETES WITH DIET

The standard American diet, often referred to as the "Western diet," is a modern-day eating style that mainly contains foods high in refined carbohydrates, added sugar, high-fat dairy, and red meat. It is a diet high in "fast food," which isn't just food from fast-food restaurants but also convenience foods such as cookies, candy, chips, soda, bars, breakfast cereals, French fries, pizzas, burgers, white-flour baked goods, and all other high-calorie, low-nutrient foods. These foods are easily accessible, do not need to be prepared, and come out of a box or bag. Fast foods typically contain corn syrup, salt, sugar, artificial sweeteners, and coloring agents, and they are mostly nutritionally barren.

When someone eats this type of fast food, it is absorbed very quickly into the bloodstream. When calories flood the bloodstream quickly, they have a more dramatic biological effect on the body. For example, let's compare 200 calories of white bread to 200 calories of beans. The white bread is quickly metabolized into simple sugar (glucose), which enters the body in five to ten minutes, requiring a rapid release of insulin. The beans, however, are made of complex carbohydrates, which take much more time to digest. This allows the body more time to break down the carbs. Beans also contain fiber and protein, which helps slow digestion, contributing to better blood sugar, increased satiety, and more sustainable energy.

The diabetes diet is a healthy way of eating that doctors often recommend for everyone, whether they have diabetes or not. It contains whole, minimally processed foods, fiber-rich fruits and vegetables, complex carbohydrates in moderation, lean protein, and healthy fats, and it greatly limits added sugar and refined grains. By following a diabetes diet and a healthy lifestyle, you can achieve better blood sugar control and an improved quality of life.

Some people might be tempted to address their health issues through fad diets designed as quick fixes that promise dramatic results. Fad diets often lead to unhealthy mental and physical behaviors, yo-yo dieting, and, ultimately, a higher body-fat composition. Fad diets can be particularly dangerous for someone with diabetes because these diets are known to increase cholesterol and blood pressure levels. Healthy weight loss focuses on the behavioral changes that allow for sustainable eating of highly nutritious foods and regular physical activity.

Making a Plate for Diabetes

The American Diabetes Association (ADA) uses a simple approach to meal planning called the "diabetes plate method." This method helps you portion your meals better for more stable blood sugar control. The diabetes plate method balances vegetables, protein, and carbohydrates. And the best part is, it's easy! All you need is a nine-inch plate. No measuring, weighing, or counting is necessary. And if your dinner plates are on the larger side, grab a salad or dessert plate for your meals.

Once you have the right-size plate, imagine a line straight down the middle, then another line that breaks up one of the half sections (see picture below).

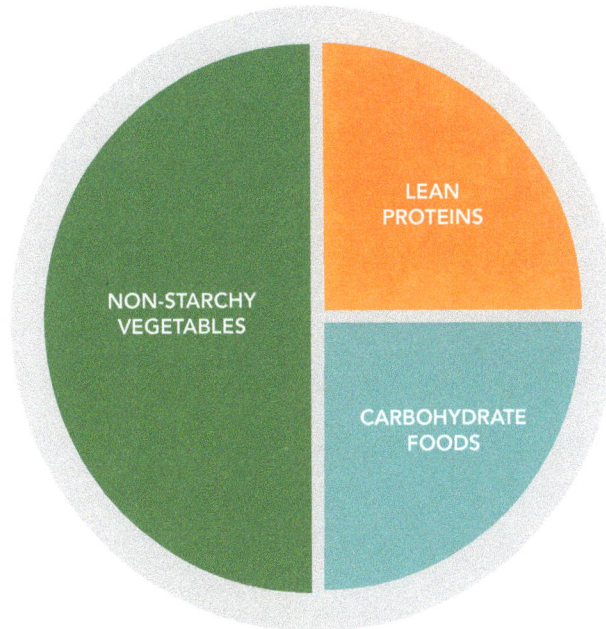

First, fill half of your plate with non-starchy vegetables.

These include:

‣ Greens such as asparagus, broccoli, Brussels sprouts, cabbage, celery, cucumber, okra, and green beans

‣ Leafy greens such as kale, lettuce, arugula, and endive

‣ Other veggies such as mushrooms, peppers (bell peppers and hot peppers), summer squash, carrots, eggplant, and tomatoes

Non-starchy vegetables are lower in the types of carbohydrates that raise blood sugar. They are also high in fiber, vitamins, and minerals.

Second, fill one-quarter of your plate with lean protein.

This includes:

> Chicken, turkey, eggs, fish, lean beef, lean pork, cheese, cottage cheese, and plant-based proteins like beans, lentils, hummus, nuts, seeds, edamame, tofu, and tempeh

Protein helps slow digestion and prevents after-meal blood sugar spikes. Protein improves satiety (helps you feel full), which reduces hunger; this is the main reason that protein can be beneficial for weight loss. Protein has a minimal effect on blood sugar if adequate insulin is present in the body. If you stick to a plant-based diet, be aware that high-protein plants contain higher amounts of starchy carbohydrates. So, if you are more sensitive to carbohydrates, make sure to balance these plant protein sources by reducing the starch portion on your plate or adjusting your medication accordingly.

Third, fill one-quarter of your plate with carbohydrate foods.

This includes:

> Whole grains, such as brown rice, bulgur, oats/oatmeal, popcorn, quinoa, and whole-grain products (bread, pasta, tortillas)

> Starchy vegetables including winter squash, green peas, parsnips, potatoes, pumpkin, and sweet potato

> Fruits and dried fruits (remember, dried fruits are especially high in carbohydrates)

> Dairy products such as yogurt, milk, and milk substitutes (such as oat milk)

Carbohydrate sources have the most significant and immediate impact on your blood sugar. However, not all carbohydrate sources are created equal when it comes to your health and blood sugar response.

Limiting your starch portion of carbohydrates to one-quarter of your plate allows for better blood sugar control. It is important to note that if you do not tolerate carbohydrates well, you may need to reduce this portion to an amount that works for your specific needs.

Lastly, choose water or a low-calorie drink.

Water is best because it has zero calories or carbohydrates and is essential for your health. Other zero-calorie drink options include:

▸ Unsweetened tea (hot or iced) and unsweetened coffee (though this often raises blood sugar, especially in the morning)

▸ Sparkling water/club soda, or flavored water/sparkling water without added sugar

Not all foods fit neatly within each diabetes plate method category: non-starchy, protein, starch. Many of our favorite meals combine each category, such as casseroles, sandwiches, pasta, and soups. But don't worry—with creativity, you can still use the diabetes plate method. Just identify the different foods in your dish and think about how each fits on a plate.

Eating to Regulate Blood Sugar

When it comes to managing your blood sugar, while the *what* you eat is important, so is the *when*. Current research shows that for people with T2D, it is ideal to eat three meals a day and earlier in the day: early breakfast, lunch, and dinner, and then fast until the next day. Eating this way, with this frequency, and cutting out the late-night snacking, has been found to improve blood sugar levels and reduce insulin resistance along with other benefits.

The advantageous effects of this type of frequency and meal timing are likely tied to the circadian system (the body's internal biological clock; the same system that also controls sleep cycles). According to a recent study published in the journal *Obesity*, blood sugar, lipids (cholesterol), and metabolism are regulated by the circadian system. The circadian system upregulates at certain times of the day and downregulates during other times. In other words, certain physiological functions such as insulin sensitivity, beta-cell responsiveness, and the thermic effect of food (the increased metabolic rate after eating food) are all higher in the morning than in the evening.

Such findings suggest our metabolism is optimized for eating earlier throughout the day. Studies have also shown that eating in alignment with the circadian rhythm—making breakfast the largest meal of the day, reducing intake at dinnertime, and eliminating nighttime snacking—further benefits your metabolism and insulin sensitivity. Eating this way improves blood sugar control, weight loss, and cholesterol levels, while decreasing appetite.

Intermittent fasting (time-restricted eating) is a hot topic in the diabetes and nutrition worlds. According to a five-week, randomized, crossover study published by *Cell Metabolism* in May 2018, the efficacy of time-restricted interventions likely depends on the time of day that you're eating. Eating earlier in the day—also known as early time-restricted eating (eTRF)—has been found to increase metabolism and insulin sensitivity while reducing body weight, fasting blood sugar levels, blood pressure, cholesterol, and inflammation. Interestingly, on the flip side, when people skipped breakfast and made lunch or dinner their first meal of the day, this produced poor results and worsened after-meal blood sugar levels while increasing appetite, insulin resistance, blood pressure, and cholesterol levels. This study found that improvement in insulin sensitivity and cholesterol levels, along with a reduction in inflammation and oxidative stress, was still seen by those who practiced eTRF independent of weight loss. This means someone who practices eTRF can see these benefits even if they do not lose weight.

That said, while eating an early breakfast and lunch and fasting after an early dinner may be ideal, you do not have to reorganize all your mealtimes all at once. Working slowly to reach a regimen that works for you can provide more benefit in the long run. Making extreme changes can cause disheartening relapses and do more harm than good. If you currently skip breakfast and graze all day and late into the evening, start by eating breakfast and reducing snacking between meals and, especially, after dinner. Also, make sure you eat adequate protein and fiber-rich foods at mealtimes so that you'll feel fuller for longer (this will naturally reduce snacking). If you need extra help, get a support buddy or work with a diabetes educator or dietitian who specializes in modifying eating behavior for weight loss and improved health.

KEEPING AN EYE ON MACROS

Macronutrients (or macros) provide your body with energy. Balanced meals contain all macronutrients: carbohydrates, protein, and fats. Eating macro-balanced meals allows for better blood sugar, energy, and appetite control, along with improved weight management. According to the Standards of Medical Care in Diabetes published by the American Diabetes Association (ADA) in 2019, data shows the best mix of carbohydrates, protein, and fat depends on an individual's metabolic goals and preferences.

The ADA nutrition therapy goals for people with diabetes have evolved over time to become much more flexible and patient-centered. Most dietitians (including me) do not offer blanket statements about the specific amounts of each macro people should eat. Instead, we base our recommendations on the individual's physiological requirements and personal preferences. If you are unsure of how much you need, work with your medical team, diabetes educator, or dietitian to figure out the macros that best help you reach your specific health and blood sugar goals.

Proteins

Protein supports body functions such as tissue repair, cell maintenance, hormone function, enzymatic reactions, and muscle-building. Protein is also helpful for stabilizing blood sugar, and it decreases hunger, making it very useful for weight loss and maintenance. For the most benefits, aim to eat lean sources of protein, such as skinless poultry, lean pork and beef, eggs, fish, Greek yogurt, and legumes.

Carbohydrates

Carbohydrates (carbs) are sugar molecules that are broken down into glucose and are the body's main source of energy. There are three main types of carbohydrates: starch, fiber, and sugar. Starch and fiber are complex carbs, and sugar is considered a simple carb. Simple carbs are exactly what they sound like, made up of one or two sugar molecules that are easily and swiftly broken down. Complex carbs are made of longer chains of sugar molecules, so your body takes longer to break them down into sources that raise blood sugar. To reap the benefits of carbohydrates, choose nutrient-dense sources naturally high in fiber and minimally processed. These types of carbs will produce a much slower blood sugar rise and are more nourishing and filling.

Starches

These are complex carbs made up of strung-together simple sugars that need time to break down. Starches are found in grains, legumes, and starchy vegetables such as peas, corn, winter squash, and potatoes.

These foods also contain fiber, which helps reduce blood sugar spikes.

Fiber

Unlike starches and sugar, fiber is indigestible by your body, so it doesn't raise your blood sugar. Fiber is good for your gut, and it slows the rise in blood sugar from starches and sugar. Fiber is found in starchy foods such as grains, beans, and fruits. Fiber is also found in non-starchy foods such as nuts, seeds, and non-starchy vegetables (leafy greens, broccoli, and eggplant).

Sugar

There are two main types of sugar: natural and refined. Natural sugar is found *naturally* occurring in foods such as fruits, some vegetables, honey, and milk. Natural sugar raises your blood sugar in a slower and more controlled manner compared to refined sugar. Refined sugar is processed from natural sugar and is found in baked goods, syrups, sugary drinks, and candy. It is quickly absorbed through the gut, and this can cause a dramatic spike in blood sugar.

Fats

Fat is essential to a balanced diet. Without fat, your body cannot synthesize certain fatty acids—called essential fatty acids (EFAs)—or absorb fat-soluble vitamins (vitamins A, D, E, and K). All types of fat are "high energy" (highly caloric) compared to the other macros: fat has 9 calories per gram, while carbohydrates and protein have 4 calories per gram.

The two main types of fat in food are saturated and unsaturated fats. As part of a healthy diet and to help lower your cholesterol levels, you should reduce saturated fats and replace them with unsaturated fats. Saturated fat can be found in plants and meats or be man-made.

All types of saturated fat are not created equal, and they have varying physiological effects on the body. Studies like one published in the *Diabetes Care* journal by the ADA in 2018 reveal that highly processed saturated fat is the fat that increases the risk of developing heart disease and type 2 diabetes. Foods high in this type of saturated fat include baked goods such as cakes, cookies, pastries, and biscuits; processed fatty cuts of meat such as sausage and pork; cured meats such as salami, pancetta, and chorizo; and cheese. While these types of foods are common and highly palatable, the goal is to use these foods as a garnish rather than as a large component in a meal. Because these foods are known to be high in both cholesterol and sodium, the amount you consume should depend on your individualized blood pressure and lipid level goals. The good news is that there are lots of swaps and healthy alternatives you can use to get flavors and textures very similar to those of these foods in much healthier ways.

Monounsaturated Fats

Monounsaturated fats protect your heart by helping you maintain "good" HDL cholesterol while reducing "bad" LDL cholesterol. Sources of monounsaturated fat include olive oil, avocado oil, and foods like avocados, nuts (such as almonds, hazelnuts, and pecans), seeds (such as pumpkin and sesame seeds), olives, and peanuts.

Polyunsaturated Fats

Polyunsaturated fats can also help lower your "bad" LDL cholesterol levels. There are two main types of polyunsaturated fats: omega-3s and omega-6s. Certain types of omega-3s and omega-6s cannot be synthesized by your body, so you must include them in your diet. But they're not equally important; research shows prioritizing omega-3 over omega-6 can help reduce inflammation and allow for better heart protection. Sources of omega-3 include oily fish, chia seeds, flaxseed, hemp hearts, and walnuts.

YOUR COMPLETE HEALTHY KITCHEN

Eating healthy can be simple when you have the right staples always available in your kitchen along with recipes you can whip up at a moment's notice. For the recipes in this book—and for making healthy recipes, generally—you'll want to stock up on whole foods. These are minimally processed and naturally nutrient-dense foods, such as fruits, vegetables, beans, nuts, seeds, and whole grains.

Foods to Emphasize

It's important to keep whole foods such as fresh fruits and vegetables and nuts and seeds available in your kitchen. That way, when you need a snack or crave a little extra something, you always have an assembly of ready-to-go healthy options.

To make a habit of healthy eating, it's also best not to tempt yourself by having the not-so-healthy foods lurking around. These types of foods sneak up on you after a long day, especially if you are tired or didn't eat a solid breakfast. Get rid of highly processed, high-sugar, and high-fat snacks, high-sodium freezer meals, highly processed meats, sweetened treats, fried foods, and chips to make it easier to stick to better alternatives. (As a side note, don't attempt to de-junk your kitchen until *after* eating a well-balanced, healthful meal with plenty of protein so you won't be tempted during the process.)

If you are on medication that lowers blood sugar or you take insulin, you may need a little stash of sugar-based candy to treat the lows. I would suggest sticking with glucose tabs or an individually portioned candy. Also, choose candy you can tolerate but don't love, so it's easy to only consume the amount necessary to treat low blood sugar.

As you try the new recipes within this book, mark your favorites so they are easy to find in the future. If you know your week is busy, batch-cook your favorite meals. To do this, make a little extra of the meal and portion the prepared food into separate freezer- and microwave-safe containers. Store them for later in the week or freeze them for the future. My favorite way to meal prep is to triple the recipes I'm already cooking. I eat my serving, then portion and freeze the remaining servings for later. If you do this with a few favorite recipes, you can fill your freezer with several options for those long days. When hunger strikes, just pop off the lid, heat up the already-portioned serving, and enjoy! Having the right foods available and putting a little extra time into prep work allows this new way of eating to become your new norm.

So, What Exactly Are You Going to Eat?

As a registered dietitian nutritionist (RDN), I feel strongly that life and food should be enjoyed. While whole foods should be the foundation of your diet, don't mentally ban all foods deemed unhealthy. Banning foods can cause an unhealthy relationship with food and lead to binge-eating behavior. For sustainable healthy habits, you need to find balance so you can enjoy life in a way that keeps your health in check. You should still de-junk your house so these foods aren't readily available. But if you are out with your family and friends and you want a treat to celebrate, enjoy yourself! Just make sure if you are using insulin or medication to lower your blood sugar that it's appropriately adjusted. Or, if needed, go on a walk afterward to help naturally bring your blood sugar back to target.

There are also times when a meal is mostly healthy, with just a few ingredients that are not. For instance, a salad with a high-fat, more processed dressing. If that little bit of dressing allows you to enjoy a giant salad of nutrient-dense leafy greens, vegetables, and healthy proteins, don't worry about it! Your goal should be to make your meals enjoyable and make them whole-food "based," meaning that most of the foods in your meals are whole foods. So rather than completely banning certain foods, I suggest a more reasonable approach. Try to individualize the frequency with which you eat these foods to your specific tolerance, health, and blood sugar goals.

One way to approach this way of eating is to consider foods in the following categories: Enjoy (~60 percent of your choices), Moderate (~35 percent), and Rarely (~5 percent). The percentage recommendations are just to get you started; you can fine-tune each category based on your specific health and blood sugar goals. If you need help nailing down what is best for you, start by eating mostly foods in the Enjoy category, then add in Moderate foods over time. If you need more guidance, work with your healthcare provider, diabetes educator, or registered dietitian.

Curating Your Diabetic Pantry

ENJOY	MODERATE	RARELY
Beans and lentils	Cakes and cookies made with 100% whole-grain flour and no trans fats	Beverages sweetened with sugar and corn syrup, such as soda
Eggs and egg whites		
Fish	Cooking oils (even extra-virgin olive and avocado should be used in moderation)	Baked goods that use high sugar, high fat, and white flour
Flaxseed		
Fruits		Baked products that primarily use white flour
Garlic and onions	Frozen yogurt	
Lean meats	High-fat dairy such as high-fat cheeses and butter	Candies (except for when using to treat lows)
Low-fat dairy such as yogurt, Greek yogurt, and cottage cheese		Cured meats such as salami, pancetta, and chorizo
	Homemade treats such as homemade French fries	
Nuts and seeds		Foods containing highly-processed oils such as hydrogenated oils or shortening
Poultry, skinless	100% juice without added sugar	
Soybeans, edamame		
Vegetables, all types		Foods containing potentially harmful artificial sweeteners such as aspartame and artificial dyes
Whole grains such as brown or wild rice, barley, quinoa, oatmeal, millet, air-popped popcorn		Ice cream
		Nitrite/nitrate-containing cold cuts and hot dogs
100% whole-grain products such as bread, pasta, cereal		Packaged convenience foods that are high in fat and sodium and low in fiber and nutrition
		Processed fatty cuts of meat such as sausage and pork

Time-Saving Tools

Cooking is always more fun when meal prep does not take a lot of time. Here are a few of my favorite time-saving tools. You do not have to run out and buy these, but these tools are useful when incorporating whole foods into your diet.

Air fryer: This is a small countertop convection oven used to simulate deep-frying, but with only minimal oil.

Blender: A good blender lets you puree soups and smoothies.

Food processor: This appliance can be used to quickly chop, slice, shred, and puree almost any food.

Glass portion-size containers: These are ideal for portioning leftovers so you can freeze, store, then quickly reheat them in the microwave or on the stove. Choose containers that are freezer and microwave-safe and use a snap-on lid.

Toaster oven: You can use this as a mini convection oven that produces similar results to an oven but requires less time.

BRINGING DIET AND LIFESTYLE TOGETHER

A healthy lifestyle lowers your risk of serious illness and promotes positive physical, mental, and social well-being. Putting thought and attention into your food choices, getting regular physical activity, de-stressing, getting quality sleep, and staying well hydrated improve your quality of life. Research has shown that the more positive lifestyle changes you make, the better your overall well-being. Living a healthy lifestyle benefits you and provides a more positive role model for your loved ones. Making these changes can be difficult, but you will see great outcomes over time by continually making small, incremental steps. Each step you take toward improving your lifestyle will also influence other facets of your life. For example, if you get a good night's sleep, you will enjoy increased ability to choose healthier foods and feel more energized to get in a good workout.

When you find a response becomes automatic, it's a habit. You have spent years forming your behaviors. So, start with small changes, be kind to yourself, and make sure you have support. When you make a change, you create new neural pathways in your brain that become deeper and stronger with repetition. The stronger these new pathways become, the more difficult they are to break, meaning your old habits are hard to shake. The good news is you can change them over time with patience, and repetition of the new habit will ingrain your new healthier choices in your brain.

Nutrition

Nutrition affects virtually all aspects of your life, and that impact is only heightened when you have diabetes. With a healthy diet, you can delay or prevent long-term complications while living a life that keeps you in control of your blood sugar.

Changing eating behaviors after years of building habits is difficult. A favorite tactic of mine is telling patients to give themselves options rather than rules. As human beings, there is something inside us that wants to rebel when we are given rules, even when we are the rule maker. Focusing on the *coulds* instead of *shoulds* with food can create a more positive headspace for change. For example, when you are given the option to eat a fast-food breakfast sandwich with sausage or an omelet with veggies, recite to yourself, "I *could* eat an omelet with veggies." That way, you give yourself a choice. Choice builds empowerment, allowing you to be your own authority and in charge of your decisions.

Stress Management

Stress is an uncomfortable, normal part of life. Even high stress from a serious illness, a painful life event, a death in the family, or the loss of a job can be normal. However, too much stress can lead to depression. People with diabetes are more prone to developing depression than the average person. Symptoms of depression include a persistent feeling of sadness, apathy toward activities you enjoy, fatigue or sleep problems, high anxiety, loss of appetite, and feeling worthless. Lifestyle habits such as a healthy diet and exercise can help alleviate depression, but, like any illness, it requires proper treatment and support. Feelings of depression make treating diabetes especially difficult. It's essential for those with diabetes to be screened for depression routinely and to treat symptoms quickly.

My biggest tip for boosting your mood and managing your stress—besides improving your diet, exercising, and sleeping—is to be open with supportive confidants. Take a moment to talk about your problems and figure out a game plan to solve the issues. Doing so will help you better manage your stress and allow you to grow closer to your friends and family.

Exercise

Adding exercise to your day is a great way to boost energy and your mood, improve physical fitness, and increase insulin sensitivity to lower blood sugar levels. When you improve insulin sensitivity, your body becomes more responsive to insulin so that you require less. Exercise also can improve mood, help with weight-loss goals and maintenance, boost energy, improve quality of sleep, increase metabolism and muscle tone, and boost immunity.

There are two main types of exercise: aerobic and anaerobic. Both types are necessary to optimize benefits in blood sugar control. The more you exercise, the better your body becomes at processing glucose and becoming more sensitive to insulin. The recommendation from the American Diabetes Association is to get in at least 150 minutes a week of moderate activity, but start where you can and work up the duration and intensity.

One hundred and fifty minutes equals thirty minutes a day, five days a week. You should also spread your workouts throughout the week to get the most consistency with insulin sensitivity.

Before starting an exercise program, get your doctor's clearance if you have any of the following symptoms: chest pain or pressure, neck, jaw, or arm pain, ankle swelling, shortness of breath, unusual fatigue, heart palpitations, dizziness, or the feeling that you might faint.

Sleep

Quality sleep helps your body stave off sickness and disease and maintain a healthy weight, lowers your risk of chronic conditions, reduces stress, boosts your mood, and produces clear thinking while interacting with others. Most adults require seven to nine hours of sleep a night. Decreased sleep or sleep quality can increase blood sugar levels. Even one night of poor sleep can lead to insulin resistance.

My tips for improving your sleep are, first, stick to a sleep schedule. Make it a goal to go to sleep around the same time each night and even on the weekends. Second, create a high-quality sleep environment. Make sure the room is super dark and that your bedding and pillows are comfortable. You should also watch the caffeine. Caffeine can linger for up to 12 hours after consumption. Lastly, while I'm a total fan of hydration, keep the beverages to daytime hours. Too many fluids before bed produces frequent bathroom trips. To reduce these trips limit drinking fluids at least two hours before going to sleep.

Hydration

Getting adequate water is essential for your body. Water plays a key role in blood sugar management because it helps pump blood, which lowers blood sugar concentration in the bloodstream. If your blood sugar is running high, one of the best things you can do is drink extra water.

Getting Started with an Exercise Routine

Here are some sample four-week programs you can use to get you started.

The goal is to increase activity until you get up to 150+ of moderate intensity per week that includes at least two anaerobic workouts.

Plan 1A: Cardio Program

‣ Week 1: walk 20 minutes a day three times a week

‣ Week 2: walk 25 minutes a day three times a week

‣ Week 3: walk 25 minutes a day four times a week

‣ Week 4: walk 30 minutes a day four times a week

Continue to increase activity per week, and start adding some anaerobic exercise into your routine (such as those in the plans below) until you get up to 150+ minutes of moderate intensity per week that includes at least two anaerobic workouts.

Plan 1B: Cardio Plus Resistance Program

‣ Week 1: walk 20 minutes a day twice a week, add two 10-minute resistance or HIIT sessions (see page 30)

‣ Week 2: walk 25 minutes a day twice a week, add two 15-minute resistance or HIIT sessions

‣ Week 3: walk 25 minutes a day three times a week, add two 20-minute resistance or HIIT sessions

‣ Week 4: walk 30 minutes a day three times a week, add two 20-minute resistance or HIIT sessions

Continue to increase activity per week, until you get up to 150+ minutes of

moderate intensity per week that includes at least two anaerobic workouts.

The following Low-Mobility Programs are great if you have a limited range of motion. Low Mobility cardio activity includes exercises such as elliptical or step machines, stationary bikes, swimming, and water aerobics.

Plan 2A: Low-Mobility Cardio Program

- Week 1: stationary or recumbent bike 20 minutes a day three times a week, and two 10-minute resistance or HIIT sessions
- Week 2: stationary or recumbent bike 25 minutes a day three times a week, and two 15-minute resistance or HIIT sessions
- Week 3: stationary or recumbent bike 25 minutes a day four times a week, and two 20-minute resistance or HIIT sessions
- Week 4: stationary or recumbent bike 30 minutes a day four times a week, and two 20-minute resistance or HIIT sessions

Plan 2B: Low-Mobility Cardio Program

- Week 1: low mobility cardio 10 minutes a day three times a week and two 5-minute resistance or HIIT sessions
- Week 2: low mobility cardio 15 minutes a day three times a week and two 8-minute resistance or HIIT sessions
- Week 3: low mobility cardio 15 minutes a day four times a week and two 10-minute resistance or HIIT sessions
- Week 4: low mobility cardio 20 minutes a day four times a week and two 12-minute resistance or HIIT sessions

Types of Exercise to Consider

The ADA recommends a mix of aerobic and anaerobic exercise (as demonstrated by most of the plans on the previous page). While walking is a great way to begin building an exercise routine, it won't produce the same kinds of health results you'll see from a more varied routine. Here are some types of exercise that you should try to introduce into your exercise regimen:

HIIT (high-intensity interval training) workouts are a type of aerobic workout that requires short bursts of anaerobic activity followed by recovery periods. This could include adding a couple minutes of jogging or speed walking to your walks—something that gets your heart rate up significantly for a couple minutes.

Resistance training can use weights or your own body. Below is a list of at-home exercises you can do for each major muscle group. Remember to rotate the different muscle groups throughout your workout plan.

‣ **Lower Body:** squats, lunges, hot feet, step-up lunges on a chair, lunge switch jumps, rainbows, glute kickbacks, single leg hops, body squat pulses, forward and back hops, and squat jumps

‣ **Full Body:** mountain climbers, push backs, high knees, speed skaters, burpees, walkouts, and jumping jacks

‣ **Abs:** planks, crunches, Russian twists, bicycle kicks, bicycle holds, supermans, flutter kicks, and lower leg extensions

‣ **Upper Body:** push-ups (wall or knee push-ups for beginners), chair dips, lateral front and back arm circles, and shoulder taps

ABOUT THE RECIPES

This book contains 150 nutritious, delicious recipes and will help you stick to a diabetes-friendly diet during your journey to improve your quality of life and blood sugar control. Each recipe includes the yield, the cook and prep times, the necessary ingredients, instructions, tips, and tricks for storage—as well as nutrition calculations for each serving to help you count your carbohydrates and keep an eye on other important nutrients.

Need an idea for dinner tonight? The Chicken Ratatouille (page 144) is packed with cooked eggplant and zucchini instead of noodles, making it super filling without extra carbs and calories. Want to try something different for your usual weekend breakfast? Whip up some Easy Buckwheat Crêpes (page 43) and add your own flare by using either a sweet or savory filling.

Every recipe in this book was made with improving blood sugar levels in mind. Look through the collection and consider each recipe's ingredients and nutritional information to find the dishes that work best for you. While there may be some with higher carbs than you want, those recipes also contain high fiber.

Recipe Labels

Each recipe also has different labels to make choices even easier if you have specific dietary needs. Below are the labels used throughout this book.

30 MINUTES OR LESS: Takes only half an hour (or less) from start to finish.

DAIRY-FREE: Does not use any milk products from any animals such as milk, cheese, yogurt, butter, and cream.

GLUTEN-FREE: Does not use gluten products such as wheat, rye, barley, triticale, farina, spelt, kamut, wheat berries, farro, or couscous.

NUT-FREE: Does not contain nuts (though this doesn't mean all ingredients come from nut-free facilities; check labels carefully).

ONE-POT: Requires only one pot and no additional cooking vessels.

SOY-FREE: Does not contain soybeans or foods containing by-products of soybeans.

VEGAN: Does not include any ingredients from or produced by an animal, including eggs, dairy, and honey.

VEGETARIAN: Does not contain the flesh of animals, including fish and other marine animals, but does contain eggs or milk products.

Tips

Each recipe also includes tips to help you navigate how to prepare the recipes, change ingredients, and store leftovers, as well as shortcuts to make the recipe easier:

PREP TIP: Information to help you prepare a recipe to reduce time and/or the amount of work.

SHORTCUT: Tip to reduce the time or work it takes to prepare a recipe.

STORAGE TIP: Lets you know how long the recipe will last and how to properly store it to help it last longer.

VARIATION: Gives a simple ingredient addition or substitution to increase the versatility of the recipe.

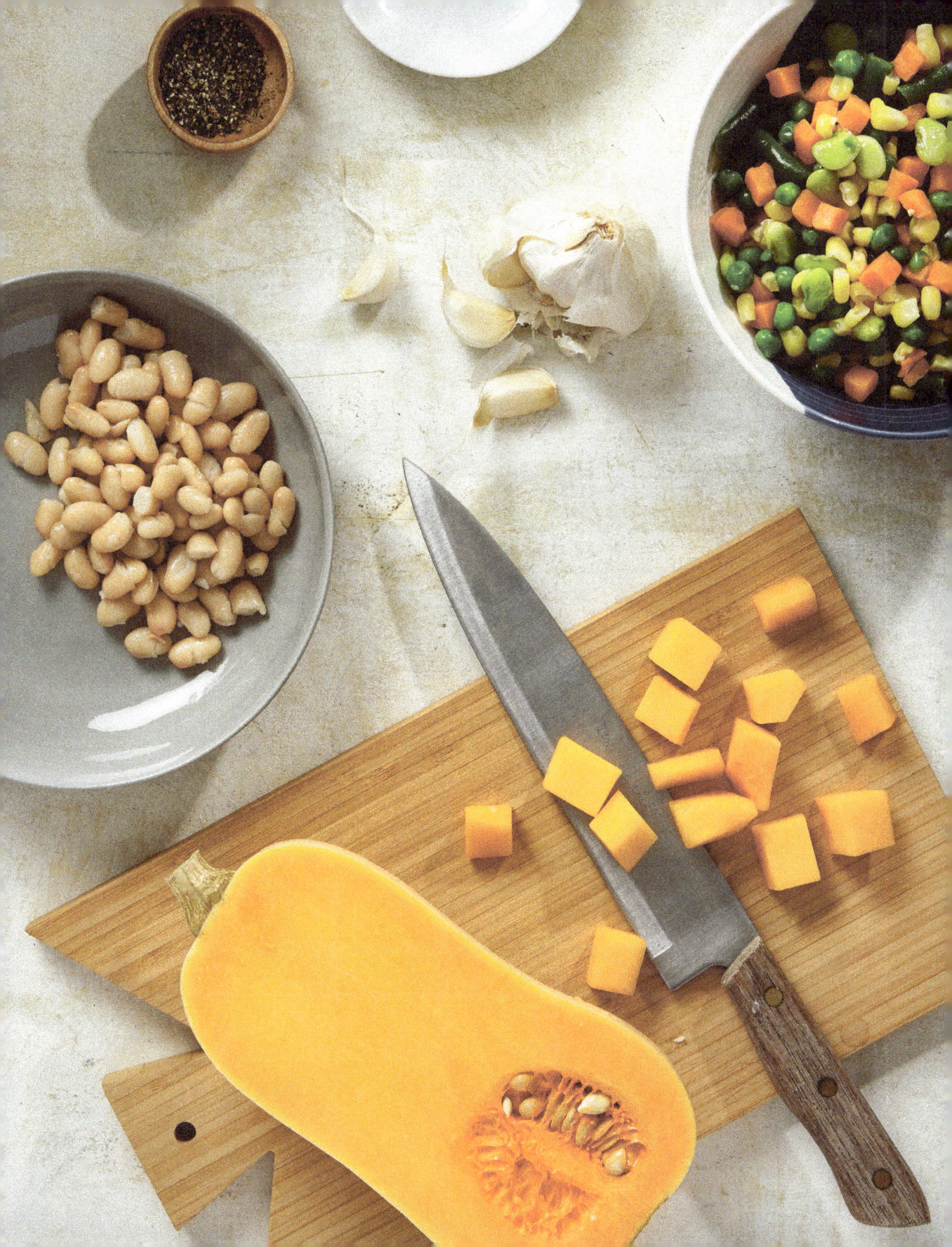

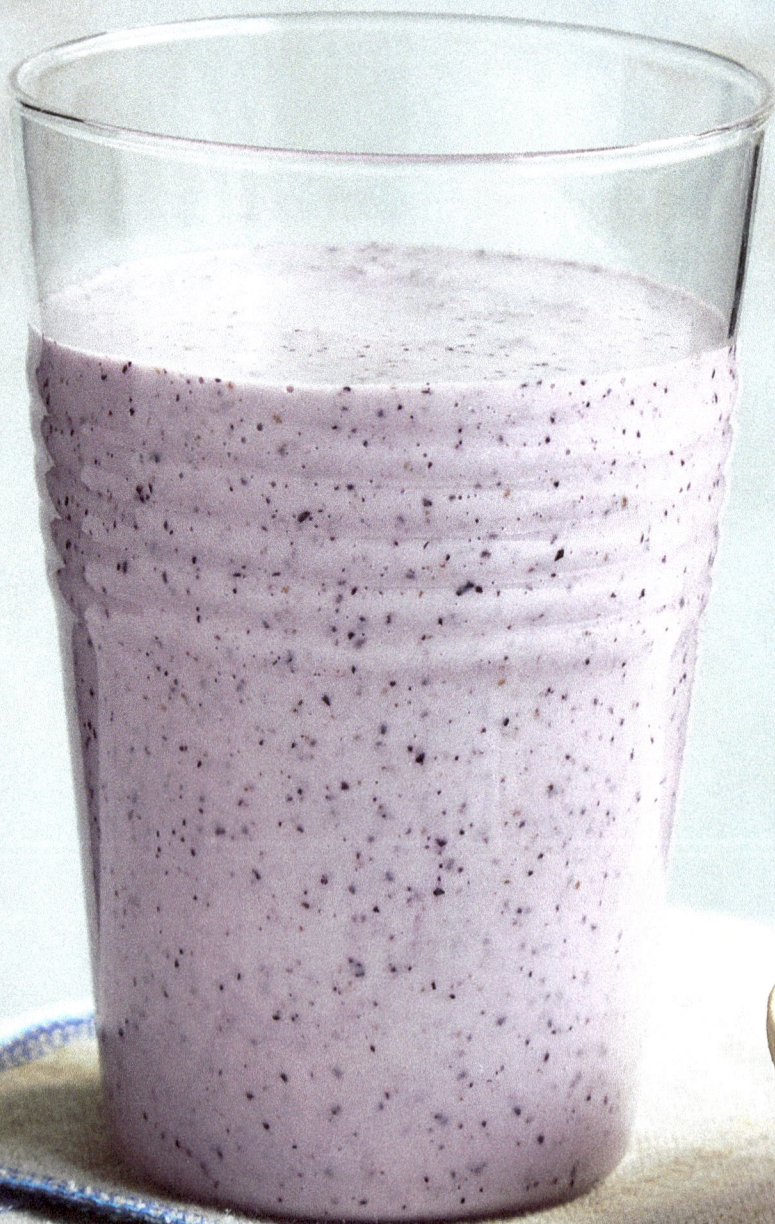

**BLUEBERRY-
CHIA SMOOTHIE**

36

2

BREAKFASTS AND SMOOTHIES

Blueberry-Chia Smoothie

30 MINUTES OR LESS, GLUTEN-FREE, ONE-POT, VEGAN

Serves 2   Prep time: 5 minutes

The blueberries in this delicious smoothie are a good source of vitamin C, an essential vitamin that also promotes wound healing. They are also high in fiber and manganese, which help the body better process cholesterol and carbohydrates. Couple that with chia seeds, a superfood high in omega fats and fiber, and you have a rich, fruity drink that is ideal for jump-starting your day.

2 cups frozen blueberries

½ medium frozen banana

2 tablespoons peanut butter

2 tablespoons chia seeds

12 ounces unsweetened nut or soy milk, plus extra if needed

1. Combine the blueberries, banana, peanut butter, chia seeds, and milk in a blender and blend on high speed until smooth. Use a spatula to scrape down the sides as needed.
2. Serve immediately. If it's too thick, add more milk or water by tablespoons until you've reached the desired consistency.

Variation:

Don't have blueberries on hand? Substitute any frozen berry, such as strawberries or raspberries. Buy them in bulk when in season or on sale and freeze for later use. It will save you money in the long run.

Per Serving: Calories: 344; Total fat: 16g; Saturated fat: 3g; Sodium: 132mg; Total carbohydrates: 38g; Sugar: 19g; Fiber: 11g; Net carbohydrates: 27g; Protein: 12g

Cherry, Chocolate, and Almond Shake

30 MINUTES OR LESS, GLUTEN-FREE, ONE-POT, VEGAN

Serves 2   **Prep time:** 5 minutes

The combination of cherry, chocolate, and almond is perfect culinary harmony. Cherries have floral, spicy flavor notes, and their pits share a common flavor with almonds. This synchronicity makes the two ingredients sing together in unison. Adding the cocoa simply enhances a winning combination, balancing the sweetness with a hint of bitterness.

10 ounces frozen
  cherries

2 tablespoons
  cocoa powder

2 tablespoons
  almond butter

2 tablespoons
  hemp seeds

8 ounces unsweetened
  almond milk

Combine the cherries, cocoa powder, almond butter, hemp seeds, and almond milk in a blender and blend on high speed until smooth. Use a spatula to scrape down the sides as needed. Serve immediately.

Variation:

You can also use cow's milk or another plant-based milk for this recipe. However, if you choose sweetened milk or cow's milk, the carbohydrate content will increase.

Per Serving: Calories: 284; Total fat: 16g; Saturated fat: 3g; Sodium: 67mg; Total carbohydrates: 32g; Sugar: 14g; Fiber: 7g; Net carbohydrates: 25g; Protein: 10g

Stovetop Granola

30 MINUTES OR LESS, DAIRY-FREE, SOY-FREE, ONE-POT, VEGETARIAN

Makes 4½ cups
Prep time: 10 minutes

Cook time: 10 minutes

Most granola is baked in an oven, but that doesn't mean it can't be made on a stovetop. Using a cast-iron skillet will create a toasted flavor that mimics the baked-in-the-oven taste. The recipe itself is written as a formula, so don't feel attached to specific ingredients. Keep it simple if you feel overwhelmed by building your own recipe; just use the first recommended ingredient in the list. Serve this granola with Greek yogurt for a complete breakfast, as a topping on a salad for extra crunch, or as a smoothie garnish.

1½ cups grains (rolled oats, rye flakes, or any flaked grain)

¼ cup vegetable, grapeseed, or extra-virgin olive oil

¼ cup honey or maple syrup

1 tablespoon spice (cinnamon, chai spices, turmeric, ginger, or cloves)

1 tablespoon grated citrus zest (orange, lemon, lime, or grapefruit) (optional)

1¼ cups roasted, chopped nuts (almonds, walnuts, or pistachios)

¾ cup seeds (sunflower, pumpkin, sesame, hemp, ground chia, or ground flaxseed)

½ cup dried fruit (golden raisins, apricots, raisins, dates, figs, or cranberries)

Kosher salt

1. Heat a large dry skillet, preferably cast iron, over medium-high heat. Add the grains and cook, stirring frequently, until golden brown and toasty. Transfer the grains to a small bowl.

2. Reduce the heat to medium, return the skillet to the heat, and add the vegetable oil, honey, and spice. Stir until thoroughly combined and bring to a simmer.

3. Once the mixture begins to bubble, reduce the heat to low and add the citrus zest (if using), toasted grains, nuts, seeds, and dried fruit. Stir and cook for another 2 minutes or until the granola is sticky and you can smell the spices. Adjust the seasonings as desired and add salt to taste.

4. Allow the granola to cool before storing it in an airtight container at room temperature for up to 6 months.

Variation:

Try spice blends to experience some new flavors. Combine the various spices listed below in equal parts to get 1 tablespoon total for use in this recipe.

Savory: Red peppercorns, fennel seeds, bee pollen

Sweet: Cinnamon, cardamom, ginger

Green: Spirulina and matcha green tea powder

Earthy: Mushroom powder and beet powder

Per Serving (¼ cup): Calories: 167; Total fat: 11g; Saturated fat: 1g; Sodium: 2mg; Total carbohydrates: 15g; Sugar: 7g; Fiber: 3g; Net carbohydrates: 12g; Protein: 4g

Seedy Muesli

30 MINUTES OR LESS, GLUTEN-FREE, ONE-POT, SOY-FREE, VEGAN

Makes 6 cups   Prep time: 5 minutes

A popular breakfast in Sweden and Germany, muesli consists of raw rolled grains, dried fruit, nuts, and seeds. Muesli looks a lot like granola but does not contain sweeteners or oil, so it is kinder to your heart and blood sugar. Muesli is also easier to make—no baking or cooking required. When creating your own, choose from a variety of rolled grains, but avoid quick-cooking varieties because those products are more processed and less nutritious. Allow the rolled grains to soften in yogurt or milk before consuming. You'll find more seeds and nuts in this than in a classic recipe; this version has fewer carbohydrates.

2 cups gluten-free rolled oats

1 cup roasted, slivered almonds

¾ cup raw sunflower seeds

½ cup raw pumpkin seeds

½ cup shelled pistachios

½ cup apricots, sliced

¼ cup hemp seeds

¼ cup ground flaxseed

¼ cup toasted sesame seeds

In a medium bowl, combine the oats, almonds, sunflower seeds, pumpkin seeds, pistachios, apricots, hemp seeds, flaxseed, and sesame seeds.

Storage Tip:

Store the mixture in an airtight container at room temperature for up to 6 months.

Variation:

Other grains such as barley, rye, or spelt can be substituted for the rolled oats. Try adding different spices, like a tablespoon of nutmeg, cinnamon, or both, for exciting variations!

Per Serving (¾ cup): Calories: 430; Total fat: 29g; Saturated fat: 3g; Sodium: 28mg; Total carbohydrates: 30g; Sugar: 6g; Fiber: 8g; Net carbohydrates: 22g; Protein: 16g

Cinnamon Overnight Oats

GLUTEN-FREE, ONE-POT, SOY-FREE, VEGAN

Serves 1

Prep time: 5 minutes, plus overnight to refrigerate

Overnight oats are easy to make; simply mix all the ingredients in a mason jar or single-serving container, refrigerate overnight, and they're ready to go in the morning. The whole-grain oats provide a healthy source of carbohydrates and soluble fiber, while nuts add additional protein. They come together with apples and cinnamon for a flavorful morning meal. Try variations with ¼ teaspoon of ground ginger or a pinch of freshly ground nutmeg.

⅓ cup unsweetened almond milk

⅓ cup rolled oats (use gluten-free if necessary)

¼ apple, cored and finely chopped

2 tablespoons chopped walnuts

½ teaspoon cinnamon

Pinch kosher salt

1. In a single-serving container or mason jar, combine all the ingredients and mix well.
2. Cover and refrigerate overnight.

Storage Tip:

You can make these up to 3 days ahead. You may need to adjust the liquid by adding additional almond milk after the first day. Store tightly sealed in the refrigerator.

Variation:

You can change the amount of oats or almond milk or even add a sliced apple, depending on how much carbohydrate content you desire. You can also top with some walnuts to add extra nutrition, calories, and crunch. A few walnuts should not impact your blood sugar.

Per Serving: Calories: 242; Total fat: 12g; Saturated fat: 1g; Sodium: 97mg; Total carbohydrates: 30g; Sugar: 5g; Fiber: 6g; Net carbohydrates: 24g; Protein: 6g

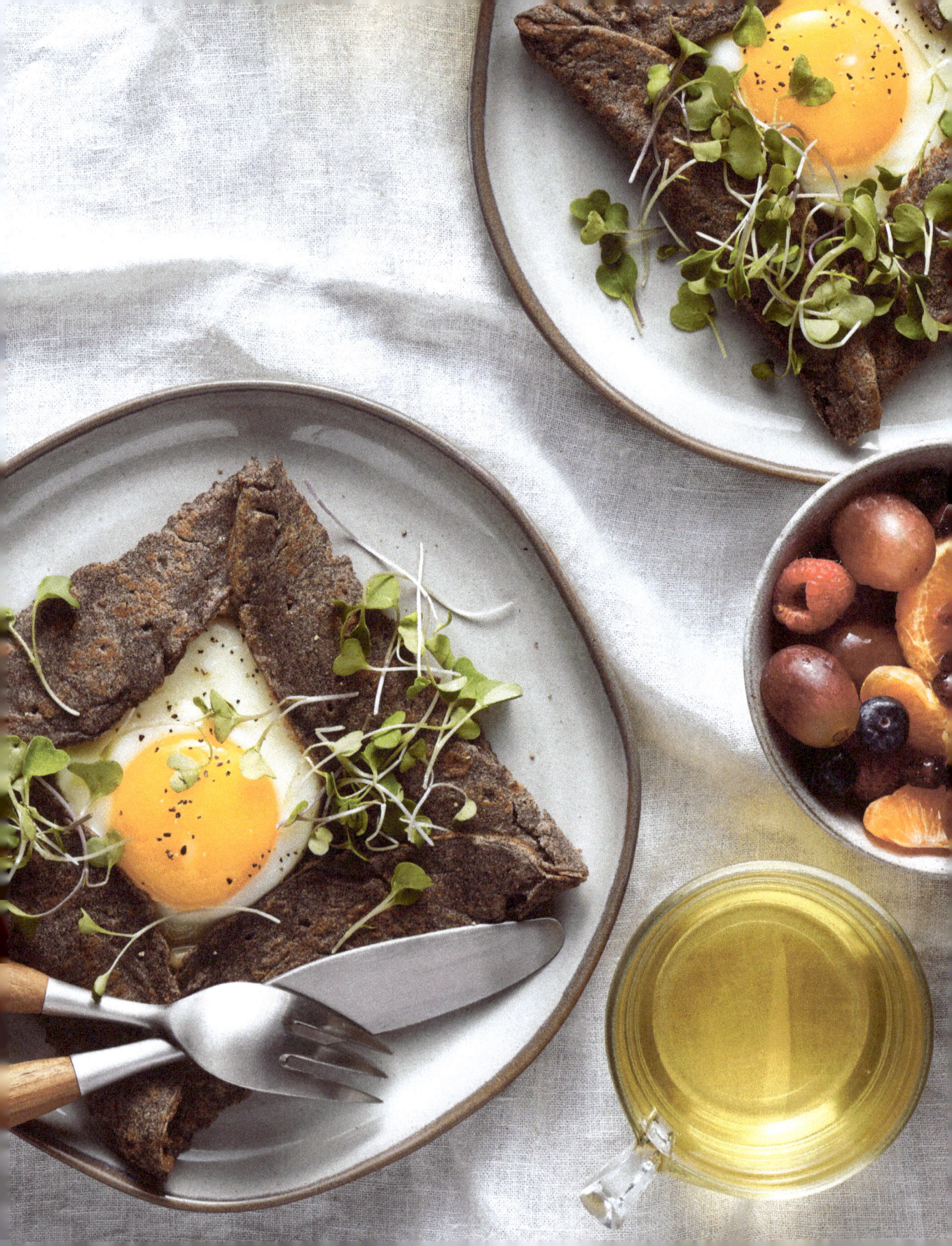

Easy Buckwheat Crêpes

30 MINUTES OR LESS, GLUTEN-FREE, SOY-FREE, VEGETARIAN

Makes 12 crêpes
Prep time: 5 minutes

Cook time: 15 minutes

Traditional crêpes are very thin pancakes that originated from the northwest region of Brittany, France. When they're made into a savory version, called a galette, buckwheat flour is traditionally used. Many sweeter versions of crêpes are made with all-purpose flour, eggs, milk, and butter. You can create sweet or savory crêpes with different fillings, including scrambled eggs, meat, fish, fresh fruit, cheese, nut butter, or roasted vegetables.

1 cup buckwheat flour
1¾ cups nonfat milk

⅛ teaspoon kosher salt

1 tablespoon
extra-virgin olive oil

½ tablespoon ground
flaxseed (optional)

1. In a bowl, combine the buckwheat flour, milk, salt, olive oil, and flaxseed (if using) and whisk thoroughly, or use a blender and pulse until well combined.
2. Heat a nonstick medium skillet over medium heat. Once it's hot, add ¼ cup of batter to the skillet, spreading it out evenly. Cook until bubbles appear and the edges crisp like a pancake, 1 to 3 minutes, then flip and cook for another 2 minutes. (If the batter starts sticking to the skillet, use a little cooking oil or spray before making each crêpe.)
3. Repeat until all the batter is used up and the crêpes are cooked. Layer parchment paper or tea towels between the crêpes to keep them from sticking to one another while also keeping them warm until you're ready to eat.
4. Serve with any desired fillings.

Storage Tip:

Store any leftovers in an airtight container in the refrigerator for up to 3 days.

Variation:

A crêpe isn't a crêpe without its filling. I recommend adding a scrambled or over-easy egg, which will add additional protein without carbs.

Per serving (2 crêpes): Calories: 142; Total fat: 7g; Saturated fat: 0g; Sodium: 64mg; Total carbohydrates: 21g; Sugar: 3g; Fiber: 6g; Net carbohydrates: 15g; Protein: 6g

Strawberry-Cottage Cheese Toast

30 MINUTES OR LESS, SOY-FREE, VEGETARIAN

Serves 1   **Prep time:** 5 minutes

This dish looks decadent with sweet strawberries and rich, cloudlike cottage cheese, but it is as light and nutritious as anything else in the book. Recipes like this one illustrate just how delectable natural foods can be, and how added sugar isn't necessary for a meal that will satisfy your sweet tooth. When strawberries are out of season, choose pears or other seasonal fruit as a substitute. The cottage cheese on the toast acts like a glue for the fruit, so make sure to dice whichever fruit you use into small, bite-size pieces.

2 slices low-carb bread (like Trader Joe's Sprouted 7 Grain), toasted

½ cup fat-free cottage cheese

1 cup diced strawberries

3 tablespoons toasted chopped hazelnuts

2 tablespoons chopped fresh mint (optional)

1. Place the toast on your work surface and evenly divide the cottage cheese between the slices, spreading it out to cover the bread
2. Top each slice with the strawberries, hazelnuts, and mint (if using), evenly distributing the ingredients on the cheese.
3. Serve immediately.

Variation:

No hazelnuts on hand? Try other nuts and seeds, such as almonds, walnuts, poppy seeds, hemp seeds, or pumpkin seeds.

Per Serving: Calories: 410; Total fat: 16g; Saturated fat: 1g; Sodium: 271mg; Total carbohydrates: 45g; Sugar: 12g; Fiber: 6g; Net carbohydrates: 39g; Protein: 20g

Shakshuka

30 MINUTES OR LESS, NUT-FREE, ONE-POT, SOY-FREE, VEGETARIAN

Serves 4
Prep time: 5 minutes

Cook time: 25 minutes

This Israeli dish is savory and satisfying and creates a choir of flavors when the garlic, harissa, and coriander harmonize with the tomato base. It manages to be just as flavorful as anything with bacon or sausage on the side, and it's much lighter and better for your heart. Some versions are green, which comes from the addition of zucchini, spinach, or tomatillos (in place of the tomatoes). Throw in a handful of spinach to boost the fiber and iron.

- 2 tablespoons extra-virgin olive oil
- 1 onion, diced
- 2 tablespoons tomato paste
- 2 red bell peppers, seeded and diced
- 2 tablespoons harissa (optional)
- 4 garlic cloves, minced
- 2 teaspoons ground cumin
- ½ teaspoon ground coriander (optional)
- 1 teaspoon smoked paprika
- 2 (14-ounce) cans diced tomatoes
- 4 large eggs
- ½ cup plain nonfat Greek yogurt
- Bread, for dipping (optional)

1. In a Dutch oven or large saucepan over medium heat, heat the olive oil. When it starts to shimmer, add the onion and cook until translucent, about 3 minutes.
2. Add the tomato paste, bell peppers, harissa (if using), garlic, cumin, coriander (if using), paprika, and tomatoes. Bring to a simmer and cook for 10 to 15 minutes, until the peppers are cooked and the sauce is thick. Adjust the seasoning as desired.
3. Make four wells in the mixture with the back of a large spoon and gently break one egg into each well. Cover the saucepan and simmer gently until the egg whites are set but the yolks are still runny, 5 to 8 minutes.
4. Remove the saucepan from the heat and spoon the tomato mixture and one cooked egg into each of four bowls. Top with the Greek yogurt and serve with bread (if using).

Variation:

If you want to keep it classic and you have access to a Middle Eastern grocery store, look for labneh in place of Greek yogurt. It's creamy, slightly sour, and cheese-like. Also, consider turning up the heat and adding the optional harissa, or cayenne or red pepper flakes.

Per Serving: Calories: 224; Total fat: 12g; Saturated fat: 3g; Sodium: 320mg; Total carbohydrates: 17g; Sugar: 11g; Fiber: 6g; Net carbohydrates: 11g; Protein: 12g

Eggplant Breakfast Sandwich

30 MINUTES OR LESS, DAIRY-FREE, GLUTEN-FREE, NUT-FREE, SOY-FREE, VEGETARIAN

Serves 3
Prep time: 5 minutes

Cook time: 20 minutes

Eggplant isn't a common breakfast ingredient, but this vegetable works well here as an alternative to bread. Crispy on the outside, creamy in the center, with runny egg oozing from the sides, this is a breakfast sandwich you will crave. You may want two, so plan accordingly if you are hungry or want to indulge in a breakfast that won't break the calorie bank.

2 tablespoons extra-virgin olive oil, divided

1 eggplant, cut into 8 (½-inch-thick) rounds

¼ teaspoon kosher salt

¼ teaspoon freshly ground black pepper

4 large eggs

1 garlic clove, minced

4 cups fresh baby spinach

Hot sauce or harissa (optional)

1. In a large skillet over medium heat, heat 1 tablespoon of olive oil. Add the eggplant in a single layer and cook until tender and browned on both sides, 4 to 5 minutes per side. Transfer the eggplant from the skillet to a plate and season it with salt and pepper. Wipe out the skillet and set aside.

2. Meanwhile, place a large saucepan filled three-quarters full of water over medium-high heat and bring it to a simmer. Carefully break the eggs into small, individual bowls and pour slowly into a fine-mesh strainer over another bowl. Allow the excess white to drain, then lower the strainer into the water. Tilt the egg out into the water. Repeat with the remaining eggs. Swirl the water occasionally as the eggs cook and whites set, about 4 minutes. Remove the eggs with a slotted spoon, transfer them to a paper towel, and drain.

3. Heat the remaining 1 tablespoon of olive oil over medium heat in the large skillet and add the garlic and spinach. Cook until the spinach is wilted, about 1 minute.

4. Place one eggplant round on each of four plates and evenly divide the spinach between the rounds. Top the spinach with a poached egg on each sandwich and place the remaining eggplant round on the egg. Serve with hot sauce or harissa (if using).

Per Serving: Calories: 231; Total fat: 11g; Saturated fat: 3g; Sodium: 234mg; Total carbohydrates: 13g; Sugar: 7g; Fiber: 6g; Net carbohydrates: 7g; Protein: 16g

Avocado-Tofu Scramble with Roasted Potatoes

30 MINUTES OR LESS, GLUTEN-FREE, NUT-FREE, VEGAN

Serves 4
Prep time: 5 minutes

Cook time: 25 minutes

Crumbled tofu is a perfect scrambled egg replacement because it's so easy to cook. The slightly curdled appearance and the added spices mimic scrambled eggs effectively. The roasted potatoes side is also ideal for some of the other breakfast recipes in this book. Try turnips, rutabagas, or other root vegetables as healthier, less-starchy substitutes for potatoes, as well.

1½ pounds small potatoes, cut into bite-size pieces

4 tablespoons plant-based oil (safflower, olive, or grapeseed), divided

Kosher salt

Freshly ground black pepper

2 tablespoons water

2 teaspoons ground cumin

2 teaspoons turmeric

¼ teaspoon paprika

1 yellow onion, finely chopped

1 bell pepper (any color), seeded and finely chopped

3 cups kale, torn into bite-size pieces

3 ounces firm tofu, drained and crumbled

1 avocado, peeled, pitted, and diced, for garnish

1. Preheat the oven to 425°F. Line a baking sheet with parchment paper.
2. Combine the potatoes with 2 tablespoons of oil and a pinch each of salt and pepper on the baking sheet, then toss them to coat. Roast for 20 to 25 minutes or until tender and golden brown.
3. Meanwhile, stir together the water, cumin, turmeric, and paprika until well mixed to make the sauce. Set aside.
4. Heat the remaining 2 tablespoons of oil in a large skillet over medium heat. Add the onion and bell pepper and sauté for 3 to 5 minutes. Season with a pinch of salt and pepper. Add the kale to the skillet, cover, and allow the steam to cook the kale for about 2 minutes.
5. Remove the lid and, using a spatula, push the vegetables to one side of the skillet and place the tofu and sauce on the empty side. Stir until the tofu is heated through, 3 to 5 minutes. Stir the tofu and vegetables.
6. Serve the tofu scramble with the roasted potatoes on the side and garnished with avocado.

Per Serving: Calories: 324; Total fat: 15g; Saturated fat: 2g; Sodium: 63mg; Total carbohydrates: 41g; Sugar: 5g; Fiber: 9g; Net carbohydrates: 32g; Protein: 8g

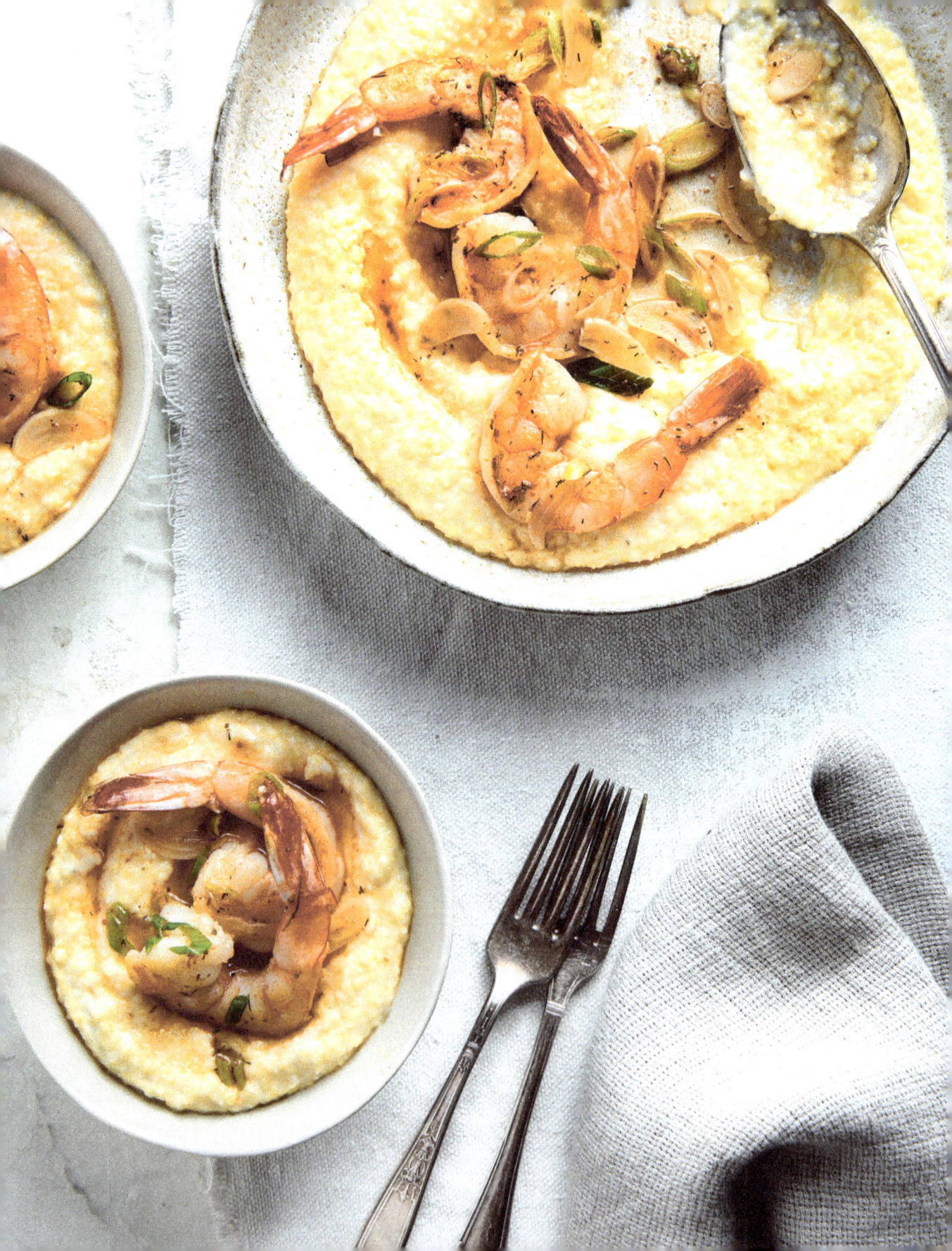

Scallion Grits with Shrimp

DAIRY-FREE, GLUTEN-FREE, NUT-FREE, SOY-FREE

Serves 6
Prep time: 15 minutes

Cook time: 20 minutes

Grits are a creamy and delicious dish, the perfect morning comfort food. Like crêpes, you can make grits sweet or savory depending on your toppings. However, this version is a savory rendition. The ingredients in this dish can be modified based on what you have in your pantry. If you have quinoa, use that for a protein-filled switch.

1½ cups nondairy milk

1½ cups water

2 bay leaves

1 cup stone-ground corn grits

¼ cup Seafood Broth (page 225)

2 garlic cloves, minced

2 scallions, white and green parts, thinly sliced

1 pound medium shrimp, shelled and deveined

½ teaspoon dried dill

½ teaspoon smoked paprika

¼ teaspoon celery seeds

1. In a medium stockpot, combine the milk, water, and bay leaves and bring to a boil over high heat. Gradually add the grits, stirring continuously.
2. Reduce the heat to low, cover, and cook for 5 to 7 minutes, stirring often, or until the grits are soft and tender. Remove from the heat and discard the bay leaves.
3. In a small cast-iron skillet, bring the broth to a simmer over medium heat.
4. Add the garlic and scallions and sauté for 3 to 5 minutes, or until softened.
5. Add the shrimp, dill, paprika, and celery seeds and cook for about 7 minutes, or until the shrimp is light pink but not overcooked.
6. Plate each dish with ¼ cup of grits, topped with shrimp.

Storage Tip:

Leftover grits can be used to make panfried grit cakes with green pepper and onion or topped with fresh fruit compote.

Per Serving (¼ cup grits and 5 or 6 shrimp each): Calories: 174; Total fat: 2g; Saturated fat: 0g; Sodium: 321mg; Total carbohydrates: 23g; Sugars: 3g; Fiber: 2g; Net carbohydrates: 21g; Protein: 14g

Breakfast Casserole

DAIRY-FREE, GLUTEN-FREE, NUT-FREE, SOY-FREE, VEGETARIAN

Serves 12

Prep time: 10 minutes

Cook time: 35 minutes

Fit for brunch with those you love, this hearty casserole combining eggs, egg whites, and zucchini provides protein, nutrients, and even a dose of fiber. If you don't have zucchini on hand, swap in one bunch of the dark leafy greens of your choice, such as collards or dandelion greens. The key is to boost the casserole with vegetables, adding volume and flavor along with a boost of antioxidants.

Nonstick cooking spray

6 medium brown eggs

8 medium egg whites

1 green bell pepper, seeded and chopped

½ small yellow onion, chopped

1 zucchini, finely grated, with water pressed out

1 teaspoon paprika

½ teaspoon garlic powder

1. Preheat the oven to 350°F. Spray a large cast-iron skillet with cooking spray.
2. In a medium bowl, whisk the whole eggs and egg whites together.
3. Add the bell pepper, onion, zucchini, paprika, and garlic powder, mix well, and pour into the prepared skillet.
4. Transfer the skillet to the oven and bake for 35 minutes. Remove from the oven and let rest for 5 minutes before serving.

Prep Tip:

To press the water from the zucchini, place the grated zucchini in a dish towel and gently wring it, or squeeze the zucchini over a colander.

Per Serving (½ cup): Calories: 78; Total fat: 4g; Saturated fat: 1g; Sodium: 132mg; Total carbohydrates: 2g; Sugar: 1g; Fiber: 1g; Net carbohydrates: 1g; Protein: 8g

Tomato and Chive Waffles

GLUTEN-FREE, SOY-FREE, VEGETARIAN

Serves 8
Prep time: 15 minutes

Cook time: 40 minutes

Waffles are an iconic breakfast tradition. This version is made with a combination of flours that have a lower glycemic index, so they are less likely to produce rapid blood glucose spikes. The addition of tomato and chive adds a savory twist, making it even easier to top the waffle with braised greens, shrimp, or chicken, as is commonly done at soul food establishments.

2 cups low-fat
  buttermilk

½ cup crushed tomato

1 medium egg

2 medium egg whites

½ cup gluten-free
  all-purpose flour

½ cup chickpea flour

½ cup almond flour

½ cup coconut flour

2 teaspoons
  baking powder

½ teaspoon
  baking soda

½ teaspoon
  dried chives

Nonstick cooking spray

1. Heat a waffle iron according to the manufacturer's directions.
2. In a medium bowl, whisk the buttermilk, tomato, whole egg, and egg whites together.
3. In another bowl, whisk the all-purpose flour, chickpea flour, almond flour, coconut flour, baking powder, baking soda, and chives together.
4. Add the wet ingredients to the dry ingredients and mix; then let stand for 15 minutes.
5. Lightly spray the waffle iron with cooking spray.
6. Gently pour ¼- to ½-cup portions of batter into the waffle iron. Cook time for waffles will vary depending on the kind of waffle iron you use, but it is usually 5 minutes per waffle. (Note: Once the waffle iron is hot, the cooking process is a bit faster.) Repeat until no batter remains.
7. Enjoy the waffles warm.

Prep Tip:

Choosing a gluten-free flour will yield a more tender, fluffy waffle. If you prefer a heartier texture, use a gluten-free flour made from beans and starchy vegetables.

Per Serving (1 waffle): Calories: 164; Total fat: 6g; Saturated fat: 1g; Sodium: 265mg; Total carbohydrates: 18g; Sugar: 7g; Fiber: 3g; Net carbohydrates: 15g; Protein: 9g

Veggie Hash

GLUTEN-FREE, NUT-FREE, SOY-FREE, VEGAN

Serves 6   Cook time: 30 minutes
Prep time: 15 minutes

This hash is full of perfectly crispy seasoned potatoes and abundant vegetables that make for a wonderful morning start. Digging into this, there's no way you'll be able to say you haven't had your daily allotment of vegetables!

2 tablespoons extra-virgin olive oil

1 small yellow onion, finely chopped

2 garlic cloves, minced

¼ cup Vegetable Broth (page 225)

2 tablespoons Creole Seasoning (see tip, page 176)

4 russet potatoes, cut into 1-inch cubes

1 green bell pepper, seeded and coarsely chopped

1 zucchini, coarsely chopped

1 yellow summer squash, coarsely chopped

2 cups okra, cut into 1-inch rounds

1. In a large cast-iron skillet, heat the olive oil over medium-low heat.
2. Add the onion and garlic and cook for 3 to 5 minutes, or until translucent.
3. Add the broth, Creole seasoning, and potatoes and mix well. Cook, covered, for 15 minutes.
4. Add the bell pepper, zucchini, summer squash, and okra. Cook, uncovered, stirring often, for 7 to 10 minutes, or until tender.

Prep Tip:

For extra-crispy potatoes, make them ahead in an air fryer. Toss the potatoes with the garlic, onion, and Creole seasoning, transfer to the air fryer, set to 390°F, close, and cook for 10 minutes. Meanwhile, in a large cast-iron skillet, combine the broth, pepper, zucchini, summer squash, and okra, and cook, uncovered, stirring often, for 5 to 7 minutes, or until the vegetables are tender. Remove from the heat and toss in the potatoes.

Per Serving: Calories: 184; Total fat: 5g; Saturated fat: 1g; Sodium: 227mg; Total carbohydrates: 32g; Sugars; 4g; Fiber: 4g; Net carbohydrates: 28g; Protein: 5g

Spinach and Cheese Quiche

GLUTEN-FREE, NUT-FREE, SOY-FREE, VEGETARIAN

Serves 4
Prep time: 10 minutes, plus 10 minutes to rest

Cook time: 50 minutes

Everyone will come bounding out of bed when you make this mouthwatering dish. Not your run-of-the-mill quiche, this recipe uses a potato crust as a shell, which provides a delightful, homespun touch. Leave the potatoes unpeeled—the skins add extra fiber and give it a rustic, hearty look. Round out the meal with freshly sliced oranges or strawberries for a vitamin C and antioxidant boost.

Nonstick cooking spray

8 ounces Yukon Gold potatoes, shredded

1 tablespoon plus 2 teaspoons extra-virgin olive oil, divided

1 teaspoon kosher salt, divided

Freshly ground black pepper

1 onion, finely chopped

1 (10-ounce) bag fresh spinach

4 large eggs

½ cup nonfat milk

1 ounce Parmesan cheese, shredded

1. Preheat the oven to 350°F. Spray a 9-inch pie dish with cooking spray. Set aside.
2. In a small bowl, toss the potatoes with 2 teaspoons of olive oil and ½ teaspoon of salt and season with pepper. Press the potatoes into the bottom and sides of the pie dish to form a thin, even layer. Bake for 20 minutes, until golden brown. Remove from the oven and set aside to cool.
3. In a large skillet over medium-high heat, heat the remaining 1 tablespoon of olive oil.
4. Add the onion and sauté for 3 to 5 minutes, until softened.
5. By handfuls, add the spinach, stirring between each addition, waiting until it just starts to wilt before adding more. Cook for about 1 minute, until it cooks down.
6. In a medium bowl, whisk the eggs and milk. Add the Parmesan, and season with the remaining ½ teaspoon of salt and some pepper. Fold the eggs into the spinach. Pour the mixture into the pie dish and bake for 25 minutes, until the eggs are set.
7. Let rest for 10 minutes before serving.

Per Serving: Calories: 216; Total fat: 11g; Saturated fat: 3g; Sodium: 630mg; Total carbohydrates: 17g; Sugar: 4g; Fiber: 3g; Net carbohydrates: 14g; Protein: 13g

Pumpkin Walnut Smoothie Bowl

30 MINUTES OR LESS, GLUTEN-FREE, ONE-POT, SOY-FREE, VEGETARIAN

Serves 2   **Prep time:** 5 minutes

Here's an easy and tasty breakfast that will provide calcium and vitamin D. Smoothie bowls are thick enough to eat with a spoon. This recipe uses nutritious pumpkin puree and walnuts to provide a touch of protein and healthy omega-3 fatty acids. Be sure to purchase pumpkin puree made only of pure pumpkin. Many people purchase pumpkin pie filling by accident, which has added sugar and spices. Remember to test blood sugars afterward to see if this healthy breakfast is matched correctly with your insulin.

1 cup plain nonfat
   Greek yogurt

½ cup canned
   pumpkin puree (not
   pumpkin pie filling)

1 teaspoon pumpkin
   pie spice

2 (1-gram) packets
   erythritol or stevia

½ teaspoon
   vanilla extract

Pinch kosher salt

⅓ cup chopped
   walnuts

1. In a bowl, whisk together the yogurt, pumpkin puree, pumpkin pie spice, erythritol, vanilla, and salt (or blend in a blender).
2. Spoon into two bowls. Serve topped with the chopped walnuts.

Storage Tip:

You can make these the night before and refrigerate them covered overnight, but don't add the walnuts until the morning. Tightly sealed and refrigerated, these will keep for up to 3 days.

Variation:

Need a boost of carbs for a workout or low blood sugars? Add half of a chopped apple for about 8 grams of carbs. If you feel hungry after this meal, try adding more nuts the next time you make it.

Per Serving: Calories: 346; Total fat: 17g; Saturated fat: 2g; Sodium: 85mg; Total carbohydrates: 24g; Sugar: 5g; Fiber: 5g; Net carbohydrates: 19g; Protein: 28g

Berry-Oat Breakfast Bars

DAIRY-FREE, SOY-FREE, VEGETARIAN

Serves 12
Prep time: 10 minutes

Cook time: 25 minutes

Rushed early mornings call for a quick yet nutritious breakfast to help power you through the day. This easy recipe is your answer. Loaded with heart-healthy walnuts (feel free to swap in chopped pecans or sliced almonds), seeds, and olive oil, these breakfast bars are healthier and taste better than store-bought bars and will last for up to 5 days. Whip up a batch over the weekend, and you'll be out the door in no time come Monday morning.

2 cups fresh raspber-
ries or blueberries

2 tablespoons sugar

2 tablespoons
freshly squeezed
lemon juice

1 tablespoon
cornstarch

1½ cups rolled oats

½ cup almond flour

½ cup walnuts

¼ cup chia seeds

¼ cup extra-virgin
olive oil

¼ cup honey

1 large egg

1. Preheat the oven to 350°F.
2. In a small saucepan over medium heat, stir together the berries, sugar, lemon juice, and cornstarch. Bring to a simmer. Reduce the heat and simmer for 2 to 3 minutes, until the mixture thickens.
3. In a food processor or high-speed blender, combine the oats, almond flour, walnuts, and chia seeds. Process until powdered. Add the olive oil, honey, and egg. Pulse a few more times, until well combined. Press half of the mixture into a 9-inch square baking dish.
4. Spread the berry filling over the oat mixture. Add the remaining oat mixture on top of the berries. Bake for 25 minutes, until browned.
5. Let cool completely, cut into 12 pieces, and serve.

Variation:

If you do not have almond flour, you can use whole wheat flour, but make sure to account for the additional carbohydrates.

Per Serving: Calories: 206; Total fat: 11g; Saturated fat: 1g; Sodium: 8mg; Total carbohydrates: 25g; Sugar: 9g; Fiber: 5g; Net carbohydrates: 20g; Protein: 5g

Egg and Veggie Breakfast Cups

DAIRY-FREE, GLUTEN-FREE, NUT-FREE, SOY-FREE, VEGETARIAN

Serves 8
Prep time: 10 minutes

Cook time: 25 minutes

Start your day with a good source of colorful antioxidant-rich veggies! The protein-rich eggs and fiber-filled veggies also help slow digestion, leaving you feeling fuller longer. Prep the veggies the night before to make this recipe a snap the next morning. Baking these individual cups in a muffin tin aids portion control, and any leftovers can be refrigerated to keep handy for quick meals to enjoy over several days.

Nonstick cooking spray

1 tablespoon extra-virgin olive oil

1 onion, finely chopped

½ green bell pepper, seeded and finely chopped

½ red bell pepper, seeded and finely chopped

2 garlic cloves, minced

8 large eggs

Kosher salt

Freshly ground black pepper

¼ cup reconstituted sun-dried tomatoes, finely chopped (see tip)

1. Preheat the oven to 350°F. Spray 8 wells of a muffin tin with cooking spray. Set aside.
2. In a small skillet over medium heat, heat the olive oil.
3. Add the onion and bell peppers, and sauté for 4 to 5 minutes, until they begin to soften. Add the garlic and cook for 30 seconds more, until fragrant. Remove from the heat.
4. In a large bowl, whisk the eggs and season with salt and pepper. Stir in the vegetable mixture and the sun-dried tomatoes. Divide the egg mixture among the 8 prepared muffin cups. Bake for 16 to 20 minutes, until the eggs are set.
5. Remove and serve.

Ingredient Tip:

Be sure to reconstitute the dried tomatoes before you begin: in a small bowl, combine a scant ¼ cup of tomatoes with 1 cup of water and ¼ teaspoon of salt. Cover and microwave on high for 2 minutes. Let rest for 5 minutes, still covered, until tender, then drain.

Per Serving: Calories: 102; Total fat: 7g; Saturated fat: 2g; Sodium: 126mg; Total carbohydrates: 4g; Sugar: 2g; Fiber: 1g; Net carbohydrates: 3g; Protein: 7g

Low-Carb Peanut Butter Pancakes

30 MINUTES OR LESS, DAIRY-FREE, GLUTEN-FREE, SOY-FREE, VEGETARIAN

Serves 4
Prep time: 10 minutes

Cook time: 10 minutes

Pancakes don't take long to make, and you can even cook them ahead and reheat (see Storage tip) or enjoy them cold, spread with peanut butter, if you're on the go. These pancakes have a nice puffy texture from the sparkling water—you can omit it and use flat water if you don't mind flatter pancakes.

1 cup almond flour

½ teaspoon
   baking soda

Pinch kosher salt

2 large eggs

¼ cup sparkling water
   (plain, unsweetened)

1 tablespoon avocado
   oil, plus more
   for cooking

¼ cup peanut butter

1. Heat a nonstick griddle over medium-high heat.
2. In a small bowl, whisk together the almond flour, baking soda, and salt.
3. In a glass measuring cup, whisk together the eggs, sparkling water, and avocado oil. Pour the liquid ingredients into the dry ingredients and mix gently until just combined.
4. Brush a small amount of avocado oil onto the griddle. Using all the batter, spoon four pancakes onto the griddle. Cook until set on one side, about 3 minutes. Flip with a spatula and continue cooking on the other side.
5. Before serving, spread each pancake with 1 tablespoon of the peanut butter.

Storage Tip:

You can make the pancakes ahead and refrigerate them in a resealable bag for up to 3 days. Reheat in the toaster oven at 350°F for about 5 minutes. Spread the peanut butter over the top just before serving.

Variation:

For additional carbohydrates, add up to ½ cup of blueberries (5 grams of carbs per ¼ cup), sprinkling the blueberries over the uncooked top of the pancakes as the first side cooks, then flip to finish cooking.

Per Serving: Calories: 301; Total fat: 26g; Saturated fat: 3g; Sodium: 302mg; Total carbohydrates: 8g; Sugar: 4g; Fiber: 3g; Net carbohydrates: 5g; Protein: 12g

Chicken Chilaquiles with Eggs

GLUTEN-FREE, NUT-FREE, SOY-FREE

Serves 4

Prep time: 10 minutes

Cook time: 45 minutes

Chilaquiles are a traditional Mexican dish consisting of fried tortilla strips topped with a spicy sauce and cheese. Often served for breakfast or brunch, they're delicious any time of day. In this recipe, you use baked corn tortillas instead of calorie-laden fried tortilla strips. This dish is an excellent way to use up leftover cooked chicken and is a great make-ahead meal that stores and reheats nicely; just wait to cook the eggs until after the casserole is reheated.

Nonstick cooking spray

4 (8-inch) corn tortillas

2 tablespoons extra-virgin olive oil

½ onion, chopped

1 (15-ounce) can no-salt-added diced tomatoes

1 canned chipotle chile in adobo, chopped

1 teaspoon adobo sauce (from the can)

2 cups chopped fresh spinach

1 cup cooked shredded chicken

4 large eggs

Chopped scallion, white and green parts, for garnish

1. Preheat the oven to 350°F. Spray a 9-by-13-inch baking dish with cooking spray.
2. Place the tortillas in the prepared baking dish in a single layer, overlapping the edges as needed. Bake for 12 to 15 minutes, until the tortillas harden and begin to lightly brown. Remove from the oven.
3. Meanwhile, in a large skillet over medium-high heat, heat the olive oil.
4. Add the onion, and sauté for 3 to 5 minutes, until softened.
5. Stir in the tomatoes, chile in adobo, and adobo sauce. Cook for 5 to 6 minutes, until the oil begins to separate.
6. Add the spinach and stir until wilted. Remove from the heat.
7. Remove the tortillas from the baking dish and set aside. Spread about ½ cup of the tomato mixture across the bottom of the dish. Place the tortillas back in the dish. Top each with ¼ cup of chicken and ¼ cup of tomato sauce.
8. Cover the dish with aluminum foil and bake for 20 to 25 minutes, until the casserole is bubbling.

9. Remove the foil and use a spoon to make 4 indents in the casserole. Crack the eggs into the indents, taking care not to break the yolks.
10. Return the dish to the oven and bake for 3 to 7 minutes more, depending on how firm you like your eggs.
11. Serve garnished with the scallion.

Ingredient Tip:

Chipotle chiles in adobo sauce are commonly found in the Mexican food section of many grocery stores. While the cans are typically small, you will have several leftover chiles after making this recipe. Refrigerate them for up to 1 month or freeze for up to 1 year and use to heat up many dishes with their smoky flavor.

Per Serving: Calories: 269; Total fat: 14g; Saturated fat: 3g; Sodium: 115mg; Total carbohydrates: 17g; Sugar: 4g; Fiber: 3g; Total carbohydrates: 14g; Protein: 19g

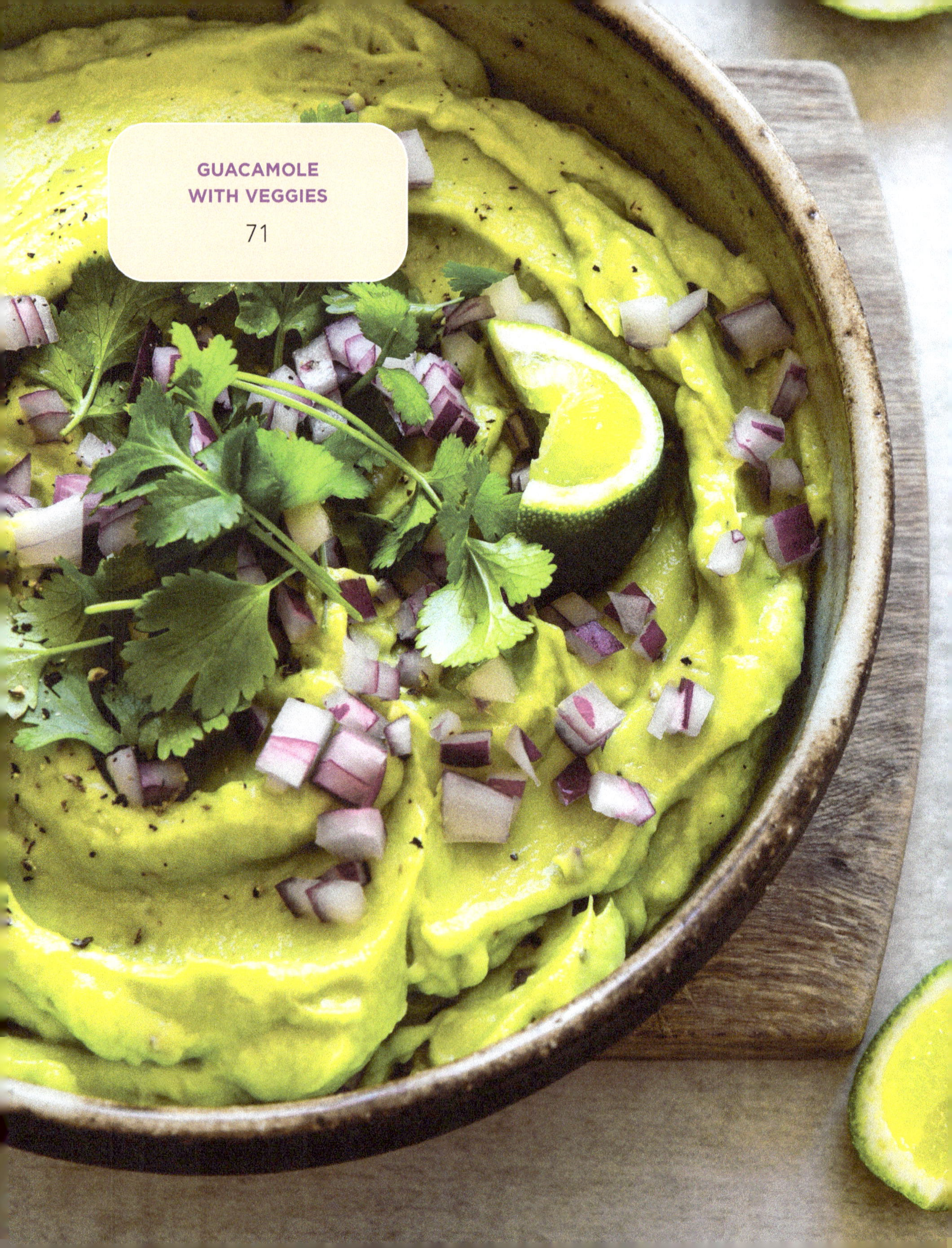

GUACAMOLE WITH VEGGIES

71

3

SNACKS AND SIDES

Blooming Onion

30 MINUTES OR LESS, NUT-FREE, SOY-FREE, VEGETARIAN

Serves 8

Prep time: 10 minutes

Cook time: 10 minutes

Sweet onions possess a mild flavor that shines in this dish. Their crisp yet juicy texture is exemplified by lightly dusting them with flour, then air-frying. Onions have been studied because they contain bioactive compounds that may have health benefits. They're an excellent source of flavonoids, a sulfur-containing compound that may help decrease blood glucose. It's no wonder that this vegetable is the flavor base that starts nearly every dish.

2 Vidalia onions, peeled

1 cup chickpea flour

¼ cup whole wheat flour

2 tablespoons paprika

1 teaspoon ground cumin

1 teaspoon Creole seasoning (see tip, page 176)

1 cup low-fat buttermilk

2 medium egg whites

1. Cut off the top of each onion, then cut each onion vertically until you almost reach the base, taking care not to cut all the way through. Rotate each onion and make 4 to 6 more vertical cuts to create blooming flowers.
2. In a mixing bowl, use a fork to combine the chickpea flour, whole wheat flour, paprika, cumin, and Creole seasoning.
3. In another bowl, whisk the buttermilk and egg whites together.
4. Soak the onions in the buttermilk-egg mixture for 60 to 90 seconds, then dredge in the flour mixture. Dunk again in the buttermilk-egg mixture and place the coated onion in the basket of an air fryer.
5. Set the air fryer to 390°F, close, and cook for 10 minutes.
6. Serve with a plate of greens.

Prep Tip:

To get the onion extra crispy, after battering, lightly brush with ½ tablespoon of sunflower seed oil on the outside.

Per Serving (¼ onion): Calories: 95; Total fat: 2g; Saturated fat: 1g; Sodium: 56mg; Total carbohydrates: 14g; Sugar: 4g; Fiber: 3g; Net carbohydrates: 11g; Protein: 6g

Spicy Mustard Greens

30 MINUTES OR LESS, GLUTEN-FREE, NUT-FREE, ONE-POT, SOY-FREE, VEGAN

Serves 4
Prep time: 10 minutes

Cook time: 15 minutes

Mustard greens, the leafy green tops of the mustard plant, have a naturally peppery taste. If you want to add a bit of heat, you can finish the dish with red pepper flakes and, if you want a tang, finish with a squeeze of lemon.

½ cup Vegetable Broth (page 225) or store-bought low-sodium vegetable broth

½ sweet onion, chopped

1 celery stalk, coarsely chopped

½ large red bell pepper, seeded and thinly sliced

2 garlic cloves, minced

1 bunch mustard greens, coarsely chopped

1. In a large cast-iron skillet, bring the broth to a simmer over medium heat.
2. Add the onion, celery, bell pepper, and garlic. Cook, uncovered, stirring occasionally, for 3 to 5 minutes, or until the onion is translucent.
3. Add the mustard greens. Cover the pan, reduce the heat to low, and cook for 10 minutes, or until the greens are wilted.
4. Serve warm.

Variation:

If you can't find mustard greens, use turnip greens, the leafy green tops of turnips, in their place.

Per Serving (1 cup): Calories: 40; Total fat: 0g; Saturated fat: 0g; Sodium: 121mg; Total carbohydrates: 7g; Sugar: 3g; Fiber: 3g; Net carbohydrates: 4g; Protein: 3g

Zucchini on the Half Shell

GLUTEN-FREE, NUT-FREE, SOY-FREE, VEGAN

Serves 4
Prep time: 15 minutes

Cook time: 30 minutes

Zucchini is rich in antioxidants and carotenoids. This wonderful vegetable can be enjoyed with the skin on, which is great news since the skin is filled with nutrients and fiber. This easy-to-prepare recipe is simple yet flavorful and serves as either a main course or side dish. The firm texture of beans combined with zucchini's delicate flavor makes for a perfect stuffing.

4 zucchini, cut lengthwise, seeded, pulp removed

1 (14-ounce) box borlotti beans, rinsed

½ onion, finely chopped

1 garlic clove, minced

1 cup coarsely chopped tomatoes

2 teaspoons Creole seasoning (see tip, page 176)

1. Preheat the oven to 350°F.
2. Arrange the zucchini on a rimmed baking sheet in a single layer, cavity-side up.
3. Bake for 10 minutes, or until the exterior of the zucchini is soft.
4. Meanwhile, in a small saucepan, combine the beans, onion, garlic, tomatoes, and Creole seasoning. Cook over medium heat, stirring often, for 3 to 5 minutes, or until the onion and garlic are translucent. Remove from the heat.
5. Remove the zucchini from the oven and spoon the tomato-and-bean mixture into the cavities.
6. Return the baking sheet to the oven and cook for 10 to 15 minutes. Serve warm and enjoy.

Variation:

If you don't have zucchini, use a green bell pepper as the base. If you can't find borlotti beans, use canned kidney or pinto beans.

Per Serving (1 whole zucchini): Calories: 149; Total fat: 1g; Saturated fat: 0g; Sodium: 25mg; Total carbohydrates: 28g; Sugar: 8g; Fiber: 7g; Net carbohydrates: 21g; Protein: 10g

Balsamic-Glazed Mushrooms and Chickpeas

30 MINUTES OR LESS, GLUTEN-FREE, NUT-FREE, SOY-FREE, VEGAN

Serves 4
Prep time: 10 minutes

Cook time: 12 minutes

Cooking mushrooms using this technique will lead to meaty, tender, smoky mushrooms that make the perfect side dish, filling for a taco, or topping for a salad. Mushrooms are rich in beta-glucan, a type of soluble fiber that is linked to improved cholesterol and blood glucose levels.

2 teaspoons extra-virgin olive oil

1 (8-ounce) package baby bella mushrooms, wiped clean and sliced

1 cup finely sliced onions

1 (15-ounce) can chickpeas, drained and rinsed

3 garlic cloves, minced

2 tablespoons mirin or sherry (optional)

1 tablespoon balsamic vinegar

2 teaspoons smoked paprika

¾ teaspoon kosher salt

1. In a large skillet, heat the oil over medium heat. Once the oil is hot, add the mushrooms and cook uncovered for 5 to 7 minutes until the liquid released by the mushrooms evaporates.

2. Add the onions, chickpeas, garlic, mirin (if using), vinegar, paprika, and salt and continue to cook for 5 minutes more, or until the onions are caramelized, stirring occasionally to prevent the garlic from burning. Serve as a side dish, salad topping, or avocado toast topping.

Variation:

This recipe is versatile, so you can use any type of mushroom—portobello, shiitake, oyster, porcini, chanterelle—to prepare it. Just make sure your mushrooms are clean! Use a wet paper towel to gently wipe the mushrooms and remove any excess dirt.

Per Serving: Calories: 155; Total fat: 4g; Saturated fat: 0g; Sodium: 216mg; Total carbohydrates: 23g; Sugar: 6g; Fiber: 6g; Net carbohydrates: 17g; Protein: 7g

Savory Skillet Corn Bread

NUT-FREE, SOY-FREE, VEGETARIAN

Serves 8
Prep time: 15 minutes

Cook time: 20 minutes

Classic corn bread has a place of honor at every summer cookout. But when you add zucchini, chives, and cheese, it nearly becomes a meal. In this recipe, the zucchini adds moisture and the chives drop in a zing while the cheese imparts a buttery finish. This corn bread pairs nicely with a heaping plate of greens and your favorite protein.

Nonstick cooking spray

1 cup yellow cornmeal

½ cup whole wheat all-purpose flour

½ cup chickpea flour

1¾ teaspoons baking powder

¾ teaspoon baking soda

½ teaspoon kosher salt

1 large zucchini, grated

½ cup low-fat cheddar cheese, grated

¼ bunch chives, finely chopped

1 cup low-fat buttermilk

2 large eggs

1. Preheat the oven to 420°F. Lightly spray a cast-iron skillet with cooking spray.
2. In a medium bowl, whisk the cornmeal, all-purpose flour, chickpea flour, baking powder, baking soda, and salt together.
3. In a large bowl, gently whisk the zucchini, cheese, chives, buttermilk, and eggs together.
4. Add the dry ingredients to the wet ingredients, and stir until just combined, taking care not to overmix, and pour into the prepared skillet.
5. Transfer the skillet to the oven, and bake for 20 minutes, or until a knife inserted into the center comes out clean. Remove from the oven and let sit for 10 minutes before serving.

Variation:

To make this recipe gluten-free, you can use a gluten-free all-purpose baking flour, which will yield a lighter corn bread.

Per Serving: Calories: 183; Total fat: 4g; Saturated fat: 2g; Sodium: 323mg; Total carbohydrates: 26g; Sugar: 4g; Fiber: 3g; Net carbohydrates: 23g; Protein: 9g

Candied Yams

GLUTEN-FREE, NUT-FREE, SOY-FREE, VEGAN

Serves 8
Prep time: 7 minutes

Cook time: 45 minutes

Thanks to the South's lengthy warm summer season, yams are cultivated throughout the region. In comparison to white potatoes, yams are metabolized slower and produce less of a glucose spike. Well-known for their deep orange hue, they're also a great source of fiber, vitamin A, and antioxidants. Here, they're generously spiced and candied. Make sure to use this as a side and balance the dish with non-starchy foods and a protein.

2 medium Jewel yams, cut into 2-inch dice

Juice of 1 large orange

2 tablespoons unsalted non-hydrogenated plant-based butter

1½ teaspoons ground cinnamon

¾ teaspoon ground nutmeg

¼ teaspoon ground ginger

⅛ teaspoon ground cloves

1. Preheat the oven to 350°F.
2. On a rimmed baking sheet, arrange the diced yams in a single layer.
3. In a medium pot, combine the orange juice, butter, cinnamon, nutmeg, ginger, and cloves and cook over medium-low heat for 3 to 5 minutes, or until the ingredients come together and thicken.
4. Pour the hot juice mixture over the yams, turning them to make sure they are evenly coated.
5. Transfer the baking sheet to the oven and bake for 40 minutes, or until the yams are tender.

Variation:

If you don't have fresh oranges, use ½ to ¾ cup of bottled 100% orange juice.

Per Serving (½ cup): Calories: 61; Total fat: 3g; Saturated fat: 1g; Sodium: 19mg; Total carbohydrates: 8g; Sugar: 2g; Fiber: 1g; Net carbohydrates: 7g; Protein: 1g

Peanut Butter Protein Bites

30 MINUTES OR LESS, DAIRY-FREE, GLUTEN-FREE, SOY-FREE, VEGAN

Makes 16 balls   **Prep time:** 10 minutes

Easy to carry to the office or to school, these peanut butter bites provide a great low-carbohydrate snack with only 2 grams of carbohydrates. Double your peanut butter pleasure with natural peanut butter protein powder (you can find it with other protein powders at the grocery store or online) and natural peanut butter. If you can't find peanut butter protein powder, feel free to substitute any vanilla or chocolate low-carb protein powder.

½ cup natural peanut butter

¼ cup (1 scoop) natural peanut butter powder or low-carb protein powder

2 tablespoons unsweetened cocoa powder

2 tablespoons canned coconut milk (or more to adjust consistency)

2 tablespoons maple syrup

1. In a bowl, mix all ingredients until well combined.
2. Roll into 16 balls. Refrigerate before serving.

Storage Tip:

Refrigerate in a resealable bag for up to 5 days or freeze for up to 6 months.

Variation:

The great thing about these is that they're small. Adding 2 tablespoons of dried fruit, such as raisins or dried blueberries, will add carbohydrates. This may be an especially good choice before or after exercise, but if adding, be sure to consider the carbohydrate count in the dried fruits.

Per Serving (1 ball): Calories: 68; Total fat: 5g; Saturated fat: 1g; Sodium: 19mg; Total carbohydrates: 4g; Sugar: 3g; Fiber: <1g; Net Carbohydrates: 3g; Protein: 4g

Homemade Cashew Queso

30 MINUTES OR LESS, GLUTEN-FREE, ONE-POT, SOY-FREE, VEGAN

Makes 2 cups   **Prep time:** 10 minutes

Making homemade plant-based cheese is a creative way to add more vegetables, healthy fats, and protein to your diet while having fun in the kitchen. If you've never eaten or prepared vegan cheese, you may be wondering what this queso will taste like. This plant-based cheese truly tastes like your favorite cheese puff or cheesy chips. Miso paste, an excellent source of probiotics needed for optimal digestion, is the secret ingredient that makes this queso ooze tangy and nutty flavors. Try drizzling this velvety queso on quesadillas, fajitas, tacos, popcorn, nachos, and salads.

2 cups raw cashews

1 garlic clove

¾ cup boiling water

½ cup pumpkin puree

3 tablespoons white miso

2 teaspoons tomato puree

½ teaspoon freshly squeezed lime or lemon juice

1. Combine the cashews, garlic, water, pumpkin puree, miso, tomato puree, and lime juice in a blender or food processor until creamy.
2. Transfer to an airtight storage container and refrigerate to cool and solidify. The cheese will stay fresh for up to 5 days in the refrigerator.

Variation:

If you are allergic to cashews, you can substitute pumpkin or sunflower seeds. You can also soak cashews or seeds overnight for the creamiest textures.

Per Serving (¼ cup): Calories: 193; Total fat: 14g; Saturated fat: 3g; Sodium: 243mg; Total carbohydrates: 13g; Sugars: 3g; Fiber: 2g; Net carbohydrates: 11g; Protein: 7g

Cocoa-Coated Almonds

30 MINUTES OR LESS, DAIRY-FREE, GLUTEN-FREE, SOY-FREE, VEGAN

Serves 4
Prep time: 5 minutes

Cook time: 15 minutes

If you're looking for a sweet chocolate delight, look no further than almonds and cocoa powder. This delicious, healthy snack is filled with calcium and protein, keeps well, and has a satisfying crunch. If you're a chocolate fan, this is sure to become a favorite snack!

1 cup almonds

1 tablespoon cocoa powder

2 packets powdered erythritol or stevia

1. Preheat the oven to 350°F. Line a baking sheet with parchment paper.
2. Spread the almonds in a single layer on the baking sheet. Bake for 5 minutes.
3. While the almonds bake, in a small bowl, mix the cocoa and erythritol. Add the hot almonds to the bowl. Toss to combine.
4. Return the almonds to the baking sheet and bake until fragrant, about 5 minutes.

Storage Tip:

These store well in a resealable bag at room temperature for up to a week.

Variation:

After removing the almonds from the oven for the first time, toss them with a tablespoon of honey before adding them to the cocoa powder, omitting the erythritol. This adds 4 grams per serving of carbs to the almonds. To keep them vegan, replace the honey with agave syrup or pure maple syrup.

Per Serving: Calories: 209; Total fat: 18g; Saturated fat: 1g; Sodium: 1mg; Total carbohydrates: 9g; Sugar: 2g; Fiber: 5g; Net carbohydrates: 4g; Protein: 8g

Guacamole with Veggies

30 MINUTES OR LESS, GLUTEN-FREE, NUT-FREE, ONE-POT, SOY-FREE, VEGAN

Serves 4   **Prep time:** 5 minutes

Finding an alternative for chips is not easy, but crunchy veggies stand in for them well. If you can find it, try jicama, because it is high in fiber and has a slightly sweet flavor. It pairs extremely well with this simple guacamole. Enjoy this tasty guacamole as a snack or pair it with meat, tacos, or fish.

1 avocado, peeled, pitted, and cut into cubes

Juice of ½ lime

2 tablespoons finely chopped red onion, plus more for garnish

2 tablespoons chopped fresh cilantro, plus more for garnish

1 garlic clove, minced

¼ teaspoon kosher salt

1 cup sliced veggies (carrots, jicama, bell pepper, celery)

1. In a small bowl, combine the avocado, lime juice, onion, cilantro, garlic, and salt. Mash lightly with a fork. Garnish with additional onion and cilantro.
2. Serve with the veggies for dipping.

Storage Tip:

You can store peeled avocado overnight in the refrigerator, but keep air from reaching it. Just place plastic wrap directly around the surface of the avocado in a bowl so no air touches it. Store for up to a day.

Variation:

Need a bit of extra energy? Replace the jicama with tortilla chips you make by cutting 4 corn tortillas into wedges, tossing them with 1 tablespoon of olive oil, and baking them in a 350°F oven until crisp, about 7 minutes. This adds 7 grams of carbs per serving. You can also add 1 small chopped tomato to the guacamole, which adds about a gram of carbs per serving.

Per Serving: Calories: 98; Total fat: 5g; Saturated fat: 1g; Sodium: 77mg; Total carbohydrates: 8g; Sugar: 2g; Fiber: 5g; Net carbohydrates: 3g; Protein: 1g

Buffalo Chicken Celery Sticks

30 MINUTES OR LESS, NUT-FREE, GLUTEN-FREE, ONE-POT, SOY-FREE

Serves 4   **Prep time:** 10 minutes

Like chicken wings? This portable version is easy to make, and it contains all the essential ingredients you get with Buffalo wings: blue cheese, hot sauce, chicken, and celery. Make these ahead; they'll keep, and they travel well. This is a great use of cooked chicken from the grocery store.

1 cup shredded cooked rotisserie chicken meat	¼ cup light chunky blue cheese dressing	1 teaspoon Louisiana hot sauce	8 celery stalks, cut into halves lengthwise

1. In a small bowl, mix the chicken, blue cheese dressing, and hot sauce.
2. Spread the mixture into the celery stalks.

Storage Tip:

Store in a container in the refrigerator for up to 3 days.

Variation:

Children might love this served on celery sticks, and adults may enjoy it as Buffalo chicken salad stuffed in an avocado.

Per Serving: Calories: 80; Total fat: 2g; Saturated fat: 0g; Sodium: 249mg; Total carbohydrates: 4g; Sugar: 2g; Fiber: 1g; Net carbohydrates: 3g; Protein: 10g

Cucumber Roll-Ups

30 MINUTES OR LESS, GLUTEN-FREE, NUT-FREE, SOY-FREE, VEGETARIAN

Serves 2   **Prep time:** 5 minutes

Roll-ups are easy to make and ideal for a grab-and-go snack. Use any wrap you'd like for this recipe, just read the labels to ensure the carbs are within your personal limit. Popular health-conscious wraps include raw vegetable versions (cauliflower, kale, tomato) and those with a base of almond flour, coconut, corn, whole wheat (lavash), or potato.

2 (6-inch) low-carb tortillas	2 tablespoons fat-free cream cheese	1 medium cucumber, cut into long strips	2 tablespoons chopped fresh mint

1. Place the wraps on your work surface and spread them evenly with the cream cheese. Top with the cucumber and mint.
2. Roll the wraps up from one side to the other, kind of like a burrito. Slice into 1-inch bites or keep whole. Serve.

Storage Tip:

Store any leftovers in an airtight container in the refrigerator for 1 to 2 days.

Per Serving: Calories: 103; Total fat: 3g; Saturated fat: 1g; Sodium: 260mg; Total carbohydrates: 20g; Sugar: 2g; Fiber: 16g; Net carbohydrates: 4g; Protein: 9g

Eggplant Pizzas

30 MINUTES OR LESS, GLUTEN-FREE, NUT-FREE, SOY-FREE, VEGETARIAN

Serves 4
Prep time: 5 minutes

Cook time: 15 minutes

There was a story once of a young boy who simply hated eggplant and couldn't stand the sight of this vegetable. What did his mother do to ensure he was getting the fiber, potassium, and the B vitamins found in this nightshade? Turn it into pizza, of course. You're sure to enjoy this light pizza and the extra serving of vegetables, too.

2 pounds eggplant, cut into ½-inch-thick slices

2 tablespoons extra-virgin olive oil

Kosher salt

Freshly ground black pepper

1 cup store-bought marinara sauce

1 cup crushed tomatoes

½ onion, thinly sliced

1 cup sliced mushrooms

½ cup shredded low-fat mozzarella cheese

1. Preheat the oven to 425°F. Line a baking sheet with parchment paper.
2. Brush both sides of the eggplant slices with olive oil and lightly season them with salt and pepper. Place the slices on the prepared baking sheet and bake until the top side of the eggplant browns, about 7 minutes.
3. Meanwhile, in a small bowl, stir together the marinara and crushed tomatoes until combined.
4. When the eggplant is browned, turn the slices over. Top them with marinara followed by the onion and mushrooms. Sprinkle with the cheese and bake until the cheese melts, 5 to 8 minutes.
5. Serve immediately.

Storage Tip:

Refrigerate any leftovers in an airtight container for 3 to 4 days.

Per Serving: Calories: 256; Total fat: 10g; Saturated fat: 3g; Sodium: 753mg; Total carbohydrates: 28g; Sugar: 13g; Fiber: 8g; Net carbohydrates: 20g; Protein: 12g

Roasted Carrot and Chickpea Dip

30 MINUTES OR LESS, GLUTEN-FREE, NUT-FREE, SOY-FREE, VEGAN

Makes 3 cups
Prep time: 10 minutes

Cook time: 15 minutes

Dips are often crowd favorites at parties because you don't just get to sample the dip itself, you also enjoy an assortment of "dippers." It is like having two snacks in one! This sweet and spicy dip is ideal for a group, but it is just as good when you're looking for your own snack. It keeps well, so make it in advance to have on hand when you're feeling hungry.

4 medium carrots, quartered lengthwise

¼ cup plus 2 teaspoons extra-virgin olive oil, divided

Pinch kosher salt

Pinch freshly ground black pepper

1 (15-ounce) can chickpeas, drained and rinsed

1 garlic clove, minced

1 red chile (optional)

Juice and grated zest of 1 lemon

2 tablespoons tahini

1 tablespoon harissa

½ teaspoon ground cumin

¼ teaspoon ground coriander

Pomegranate arils (seeds) (optional)

Cilantro, chopped (optional)

1. Preheat the oven to 425°F. Line a baking sheet with parchment paper.
2. In a medium bowl, toss the carrots with 2 teaspoons of olive oil, salt, and pepper. Spread them in a single layer on the prepared baking sheet and roast until tender, tossing halfway through, about 15 minutes.
3. Meanwhile, place the chickpeas, garlic, chile (if using), lemon juice, lemon zest, tahini, harissa, cumin, and coriander in a food processor. Set aside. Add the carrots to the processor when they are cooked. Pulse until the mixture is coarse. Scrape the bowl down, then turn the processor back on while you drizzle the remaining ¼ cup of olive oil through the feed tube of the machine. Adjust the seasonings as desired. If it's too thick, add water to thin.
4. Top with pomegranate arils and chopped cilantro (if using), and serve with cut vegetables.

Variation:

Use tomato paste instead of harissa if you don't have it ready or if you want less spice.

Per Serving (¼ cup): Calories: 105; Total fat: 7g; Saturated fat: 1g; Sodium: 32mg; Total carbohydrates: 8g; Sugar: 2g; Fiber: 2g; Net carbohydrates: 6g; Protein: 2g

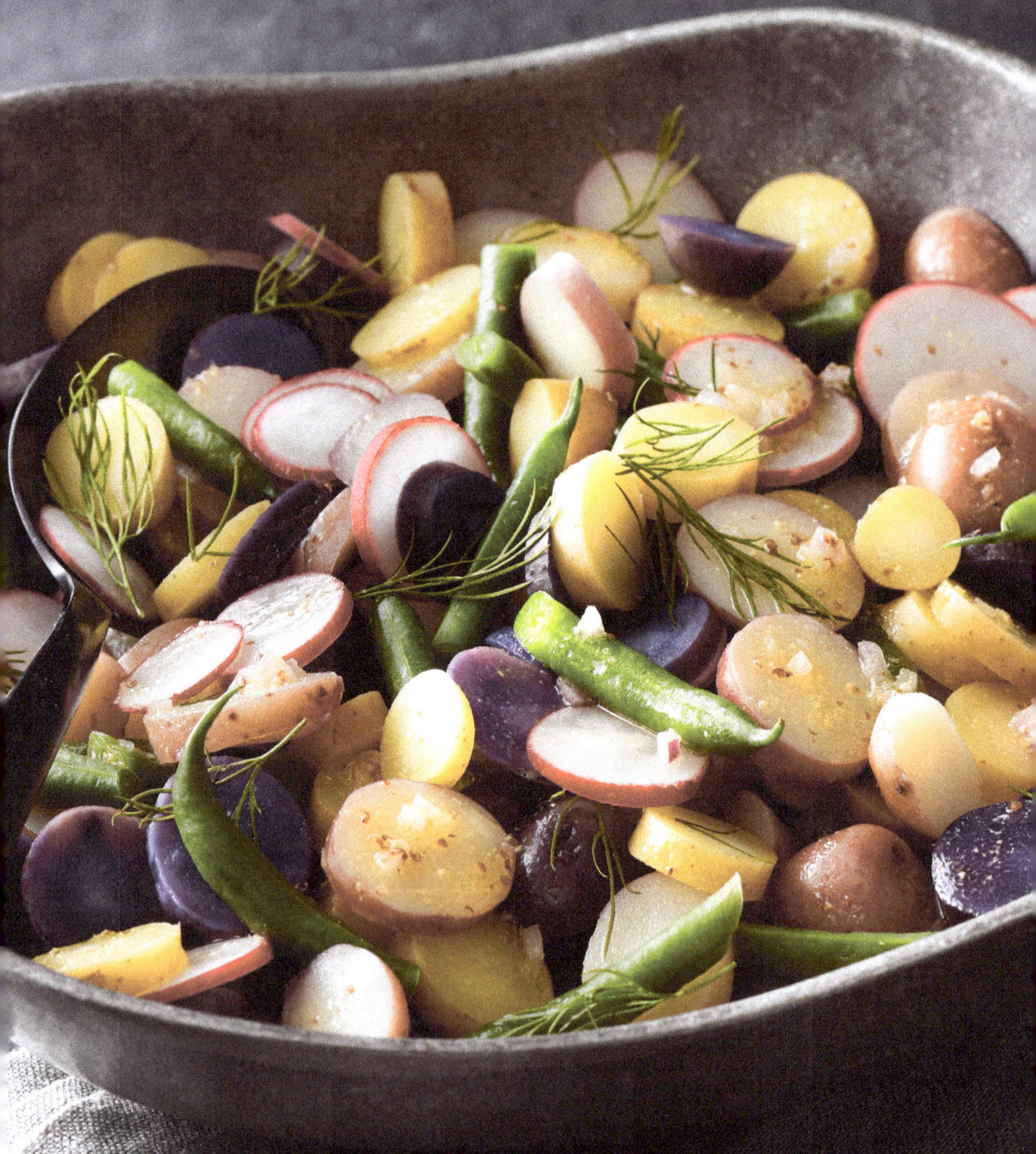

Green Bean and Radish Potato Salad

30 MINUTES OR LESS, GLUTEN-FREE, NUT-FREE, SOY-FREE, VEGAN

Serves 6
Prep time: 10 minutes

Cook time: 20 minutes

Fingerling potatoes—those small multicolored potatoes similar in size to fingers (hence their name)—have a robust, earthy, and buttery flavor. They are wonderful in salads, because they keep their shape after cooking due to their firmness. If you cannot find fingerlings, Yukon Gold potatoes will also work in this recipe.

Kosher salt

6 ounces fresh green beans, trimmed and cut into 1-inch pieces

1½ pounds fingerling potatoes

⅓ cup extra-virgin olive oil

2 tablespoons freshly squeezed lemon juice

1 tablespoon Dijon or whole-grain mustard

1 shallot, minced

8 radishes, thinly sliced

¼ cup fresh dill, chopped

Freshly ground black pepper

1. Place a small saucepan filled three-quarters full of water and a pinch of salt over high heat and bring it to a boil. Add the green beans and boil for 2 minutes, then transfer them with a slotted spoon to a colander. Run the beans under cold running water until cool and transfer to a medium bowl.
2. Place the potatoes in the same pot of boiling water, reduce the heat to low, and simmer until tender, about 12 minutes.
3. Meanwhile, combine the olive oil, lemon juice, mustard, and shallot in a jar. Seal with the lid and shake vigorously. If you don't have a jar with a fitted lid, you can also whisk the ingredients in a bowl.
4. Transfer the cooked potatoes to a colander and cool them under cold running water. When they're cool enough to handle, slice the potatoes into thin rounds.
5. Add the potatoes and dressing to the bowl with the green beans, along with the radishes and dill, and toss to combine.
6. Season with salt and pepper and serve.

Storage Tip:

Refrigerate any leftovers in an airtight container for 3 to 4 days.

Per Serving: Calories: 208; Total fat: 12g; Saturated fat: 2g; Sodium: 66mg; Total carbohydrates: 24g; Sugar: 2g; Fiber: 3g; Net carbohydrates: 21g; Protein: 3g

Charred Sesame Broccoli

30 MINUTES OR LESS, GLUTEN-FREE, NUT-FREE, VEGAN

Serves 4
Prep time: 5 minutes

Cook time: 15 minutes

Broccoli is ubiquitous, but often people overcook it until it's army green in color and turns to mush. This is highly undesirable in both appearance and flavor. Try cooking your broccoli using this method, and you'll have everyone reaching for it. Broccoli is loaded with fiber, calcium, folate, potassium, and iron and supports bone health, brain function, and heart health.

1 tablespoon
   extra-virgin olive oil

1 tablespoon
   reduced-sodium
   soy sauce

½ tablespoon
   sesame oil

1 head broccoli, cut
   into florets

1 tablespoon toasted
   sesame seeds

1. Preheat the oven to 450°F. Line a baking sheet with parchment paper.
2. In a medium bowl, whisk together the olive oil, soy sauce, and sesame oil. Add the broccoli and toss to evenly coat it.
3. Spread the coated broccoli on the prepared baking sheet and bake for 10 minutes, until tender.
4. Remove the sheet from the oven, flip the broccoli over, and return it to the oven for an additional 5 to 10 minutes.
5. Serve the broccoli with toasted sesame seeds on top.

Storage Tip:

Refrigerate any leftovers in an airtight container for up to 4 days.

Variation:

You can use regular broccoli here, but also give Chinese broccoli a try if it's available. Called *gai lan*, it is one of the most popular greens in all of China and has a stronger, slightly bitter note that lends itself well to the sesame and the soy of this dish. Broccoli rabe is also an inspired choice.

Per Serving: Calories: 110; Total fat: 7g; Saturated fat: 1g; Sodium: 185mg; Total carbohydrates: 11g; Sugar: 2g; Fiber: 4g; Net carbohydrates: 7g; Protein: 5g

Smashed Cucumber Salad

30 MINUTES OR LESS, GLUTEN-FREE, NUT-FREE, SOY-FREE, VEGAN

Serves 4   **Prep time:** 10 minutes

Smashing cucumbers for a salad is a standard technique in many parts of Asia. Once you've tried it, you'll understand why it's such a great idea, and not just for taking out your aggression. Smashing a cucumber changes the way it picks up the flavors. More cucumber cells open and allow for some water to escape, while absorbing other added ingredients, thus changing the overall taste.

2 pounds mini cucumbers (English or Persian), unpeeled

½ teaspoon kosher salt

1 tablespoon extra-virgin olive oil

¾ teaspoon ground cumin

¼ teaspoon turmeric

Juice of 1 lime

½ cup cilantro leaves

1. Cut the cucumbers crosswise into 4-inch pieces and again in half lengthwise.
2. On a work surface, place one cucumber flesh-side down. Place the side of the knife blade on the cucumber and carefully smash down lightly with your hand. Alternatively, put in a plastic bag, seal, and smash with a rolling pin or similar tool. Be careful not to break the bag. The skin of the cucumber should crack, and flesh will break away. Repeat with all the cucumbers and cut the smashed pieces on a bias into bite-size pieces.
3. Transfer the cucumber pieces to a strainer and toss them with the salt. Allow the cucumbers to rest for at least 15 minutes.
4. Meanwhile, prepare the dressing. In a small bowl, whisk together the olive oil, cumin, turmeric, and lime juice.
5. When the cucumbers are ready, shake them to remove any excess liquid. Transfer the cucumbers to a large bowl with the dressing and cilantro and toss to combine. Serve.

Ingredient Tip:

Use fresh, firm-fleshed cucumbers and avoid those that are older and soft. Your standard greenhouse variety commonly found in grocery stores will work just fine but is best when the seeds are removed before it's smashed.

Per Serving: Calories: 69; Total fat: 4g; Saturated fat: 0g; Sodium: 152mg; Total carbohydrates: 10g; Sugar: 4g; Fiber: 2g; Net carbohydrates: 8g; Protein: 2g

Roasted Asparagus with Romesco Sauce

30 MINUTES OR LESS, SOY-FREE, VEGAN

Serves 2
Prep time: 5 minutes

Cook time: 15 minutes

Asparagus is one of the true harbingers of warm weather, along with the birdsongs and delicate budding flowers, of course. Romesco sauce brings out the natural, earthy flavor of the asparagus and adds a punch of its own to create a perfect balance. You can roast or grill the asparagus—both are equally tasty.

1 bunch
asparagus, woody
ends removed

1 tablespoon
extra-virgin olive oil

¼ to ½ cup Romesco
Sauce (page 81) or
store-bought

Roasted method

1. Preheat the oven to 425°F. Line a baking sheet with parchment paper.
2. In a medium bowl, toss the asparagus with the olive oil.
3. Place the asparagus on the baking sheet and roast until tender, 12 to 15 minutes.
4. Remove the asparagus from the heat, arrange it on a serving platter, top it with romesco sauce, and serve.

Grill method

1. Preheat the grill to high heat.
2. In a medium bowl, toss the asparagus with the olive oil.
3. Place the asparagus on a grill pan or directly on the grill grates and sear for 2 to 4 minutes until tender, turning them as often as you need to avoid burning.
4. Remove the asparagus from the heat, arrange it on a serving platter, top it with romesco sauce, and serve.

Storage Tip:

Refrigerate any leftovers in an airtight container for 3 to 4 days.

Per Serving: Calories: 110; Total fat: 8g; Saturated fat: 1g; Sodium: 550mg; Total carbohydrates: 7g; Sugar: 2g; Fiber: 5g; Net carbohydrates: 2g; Protein: 7g

Romesco Sauce

Makes ~2 cups

Prep time: 5 to 10 minutes

3 roasted red
  bell peppers

2 slices toasted whole
  wheat bread, cubed

1 medium tomato

5 garlic cloves

½ cup toasted almonds

2 tablespoons
  sherry vinegar

1 tablespoon
  smoked paprika

¼ teaspoon kosher salt

¼ teaspoon
  cayenne pepper

¼ cup extra-virgin
  olive oil

In a food processor, combine the bell peppers, bread, tomato, garlic, almonds, sherry vinegar, paprika, salt, and cayenne. Puree, then, while the machine is running, slowly stream in the olive oil. Stop the machine, taste, and adjust the seasonings as desired. Refrigerate in an airtight container for up to 1 week or freeze for up to 3 months.

Per Serving (½ cup): Calories: 310; Total fat: 24g; Saturated fat: 3g; Sodium: 285mg; Total carbohydrates: 19g; Sugar: 5g; Fiber: 5g; Net carbohydrates: 14g; Protein: 8g

Kale Chip Nachos

30 MINUTES OR LESS, GLUTEN-FREE, NUT-FREE, SOY-FREE, VEGAN

Serves 3　　　　　　　　　　　　　　　**Cook time:** 20 minutes
Prep time: 10 minutes

When you're looking for something to snack on while watching the game or your favorite show, you want to make sure it's something nutritious, but, even better, gives you a tasty crunch. This version of nachos uses kale as the base, so you can snack away while getting the nutritional boost that comes from this hearty green alongside sweet potato and black beans.

1 bunch kale, torn into bite-size pieces	2 teaspoons ground cumin, divided	1 (15-ounce) can low-sodium black beans, drained and rinsed	½ teaspoon ground coriander
3 tablespoons extra-virgin olive oil, divided	1 large sweet potato, cut into ¼-inch-thick rounds		1 teaspoon chili powder

Optional toppings

Avocado slices	Jicama, sliced	Fresh cilantro	Fresh tomatoes, diced
Salsa	Red onion, sliced	Fresh chiles, minced	

1. Preheat the oven to 225°F. Line a baking sheet with parchment paper.
2. In a large bowl, toss the kale with 1 tablespoon of olive oil and 1 teaspoon of cumin. Use your hands to massage the kale and evenly distribute the oil.
3. Spread the kale in a single even layer on the prepared baking sheet. (You may need two lined baking sheets for this.) Bake for 15 minutes, then flip and toss, and bake for another 5 to 10 minutes.
4. Meanwhile, heat 1 tablespoon of oil in a large skillet over medium-high heat. Arrange the sweet potato rounds in a single layer in the skillet, cover, and let them cook until they begin to brown on the bottom, about 3 minutes. Flip the potatoes over and cook for 3 to 5 minutes more.
5. Add the black beans to the skillet with the remaining 1 tablespoon of oil, the remaining 1 teaspoon of cumin, the coriander, and the chili powder. Cook for 3 minutes, then set aside and keep warm if the kale is not yet finished baking.
6. Serve on a platter, starting with the kale as a base, topped with sweet potatoes, black beans, and finally, any optional toppings.

Storage Tip:

Refrigerate any leftovers in an airtight container for 3 to 4 days.

Variation:

You can use any kind of canned beans or lentils in place of the black beans for additional variety with this recipe.

Per Serving: Calories: 288; Total fat: 13g; Saturated fat: 2g; Sodium: 162mg; Total carbohydrates: 32g; Sugar: 2g; Fiber: 10g; Net carbohydrates: 22g; Protein: 10g

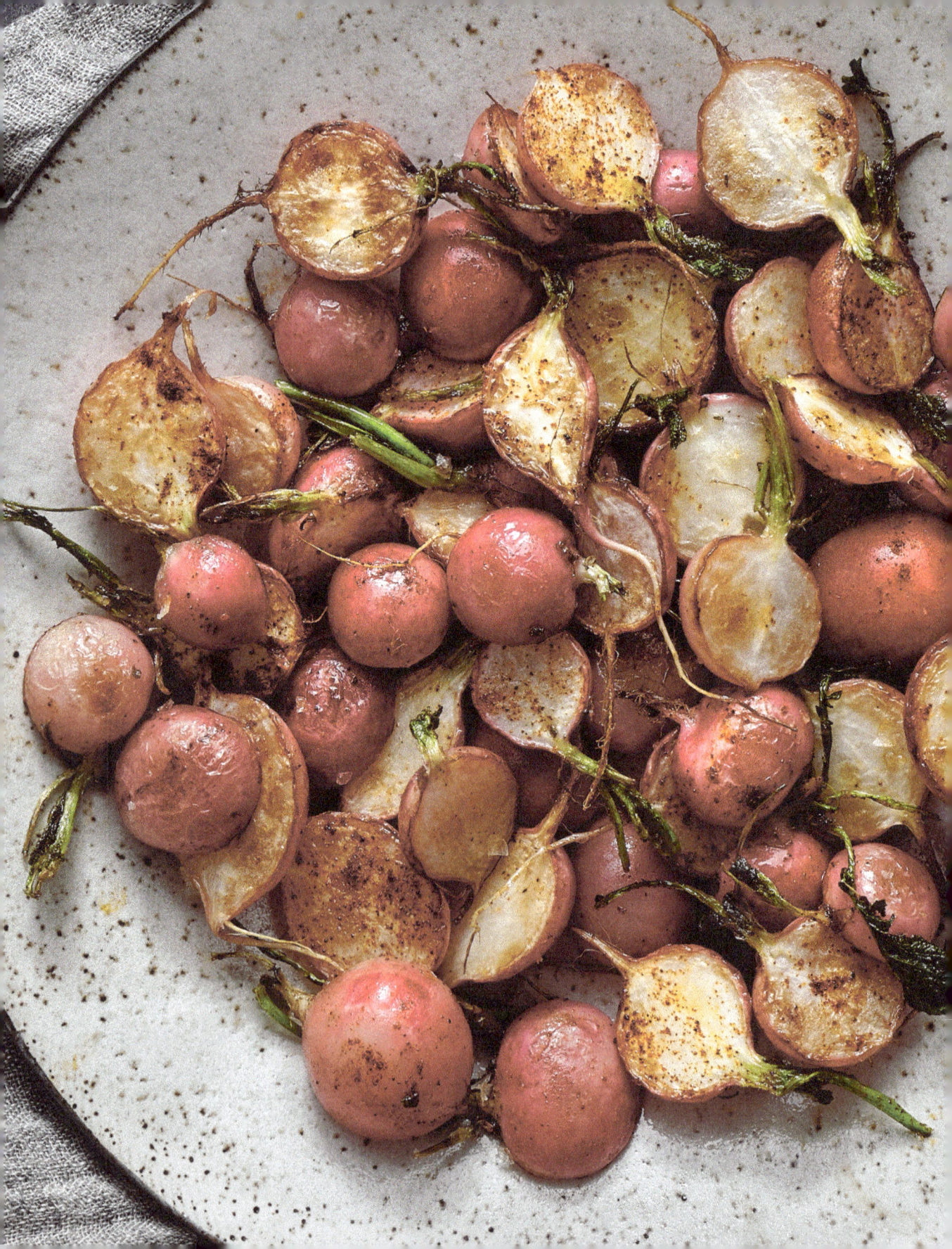

Garlic-Roasted Radishes

30 MINUTES OR LESS, GLUTEN-FREE, NUT-FREE, SOY-FREE, VEGAN

Serves 2
Prep time: 5 minutes

Cook time: 15 minutes

Radishes are one of spring's greatest treats. They are cruciferous, like broccoli and cabbage, which means they have many of the same cancer-fighting compounds as these powerhouse vegetables. They also have a positive impact on the fight against diabetes, as some studies suggest eating radishes may help improve blood sugar control. Radishes are also delicious and come in a multitude of colors that look great on the plate.

1 pound radishes, halved	1 tablespoon avocado oil	4 garlic cloves, thinly sliced	¼ cup chopped fresh dill
	Pinch kosher salt		

1. Preheat the oven to 425°F. Line a baking sheet with parchment paper.
2. In a medium bowl, toss the radishes with the avocado oil and salt. Spread the radishes on the prepared baking sheet and roast for 10 minutes. Remove the sheet from the oven, add the garlic, mix well, and return to the oven for 5 minutes.
3. Remove the radishes from the oven, adjust the seasoning as desired, and serve topped with dill on a serving plate or as a side dish.

Storage Tip:

Store any leftovers in an airtight container in the refrigerator for 3 to 4 days.

Variation:

For a different flavor profile, swap out the fresh dill garnish for a squeeze of lime juice, a dusting of paprika, and a pinch of chili powder.

Per Serving: Calories: 110; Total fat: 7g; Saturated fat: 1g; Sodium: 168mg; Total carbohydrates: 10g; Sugar: 4g; Fiber: 4g; Net carbohydrates: 6g; Protein: 2g

FIRST-OF-THE-SEASON TOMATO, PEACH, AND STRAWBERRY SALAD

91

4

SOUPS, SALADS, AND SANDWICHES

Roasted Tomato Tartine

30 MINUTES OR LESS, NUT-FREE, SOY-FREE, VEGETARIAN

Serves 2
Prep time: 5 minutes

Cook time: 15 minutes

Less bread, more tomato is the equation for this delicious sandwich. This recipe goes to show that you don't have to remove bread entirely from your diet; instead, just don't eat as much. Flavorful whole-grain bread acts as a vehicle here for vibrant tomatoes, fresh basil, and tart balsamic vinegar. If you want to add more seasonings or fresh herbs, it's up to you.

- 3 tomatoes, cut into eighths
- 2 tablespoons extra-virgin olive oil, divided
- 1 tablespoon balsamic vinegar
- 2 garlic cloves, minced
- Pinch kosher salt
- Pinch freshly ground black pepper
- ½ cup nonfat cottage cheese
- 2 slices whole-grain bread
- 2 tablespoons chopped fresh basil
- 4 cups arugula

1. Preheat the oven to 450°F. Line a baking sheet with parchment paper.
2. In a medium-size bowl, toss the tomatoes with 1 tablespoon of olive oil, the vinegar, the garlic, salt, and pepper.
3. Spread the tomatoes on the baking sheet and bake for 15 minutes.
4. Meanwhile, place the cottage cheese in the bowl of a food processor and, while it is running, add the remaining 1 tablespoon of olive oil in a thin stream. Pause to scrape down the sides if needed. Taste and adjust the seasonings as needed. If you do not have a food processor, whisk the cottage cheese and olive oil in a medium bowl.
5. Toast the bread and divide the cottage cheese between the slices, spreading it out evenly. Top the cottage cheese with the tomatoes and garnish with chopped basil.
6. Serve with the arugula on the side.

Variation:

Want more cheese whip on this sandwich? Double it up on the bread or double it anyway and store the extra in the refrigerator for up to 1 week for other recipes. Adjust the seasonings with freshly ground black pepper for an even better flavor.

Per Serving: Calories: 270; Total fat: 15g; Saturated fat: 2g; Sodium: 334mg; Total carbohydrates: 24g; Sugar: 9g; Fiber: 5g; Net carbohydrates: 19g; Protein: 10g

Cauli-Lettuce Wraps

30 MINUTES OR LESS, ONE-POT, VEGAN

Serves 4
Prep time: 10 minutes

Cook time: 20 minutes

This is a low-calorie, low-carbohydrate meal that will leave your body feeling refreshed and light. With lots of flavor and crunch, it makes for a satisfying meal that's just what the dietitian ordered to keep your blood sugar on track.

- 1½ tablespoons sesame oil
- ½ yellow onion, chopped
- 8 ounces mushrooms, thinly sliced
- 4 garlic cloves, minced

- 1½ tablespoons reduced-sodium soy sauce or tamari
- 4 teaspoons rice wine vinegar
- 5 ounces water chestnuts, drained and liquid reserved

- 2½ cups Cauliflower Rice (page 213)
- ½ cup coarsely chopped cashews
- 4 large green leaf lettuce leaves

- 2 scallions, both white and green parts, thinly sliced (optional)
- 1 cup chopped cilantro (optional)

1. In a large skillet over medium heat, heat the sesame oil and sauté the onion until translucent, about 3 minutes. Add the mushrooms, garlic, tamari, vinegar, and water chestnuts to the skillet. Cover the skillet with a lid and cook until the mushrooms are softened, about 5 minutes.
2. Add the cauliflower rice and cashews and mix well. Cover the skillet and cook for 2 minutes.
3. Adjust the seasonings as desired and evenly divide the cauliflower mixture among the lettuce leaves.
4. Serve garnished with scallions (if using) and cilantro (if using).

Storage Tip:

Refrigerate any leftovers in an airtight container for up to 2 days.

Variation:

Use white vinegar or mirin if you can't find rice wine vinegar. Add a fresh chile or some chili oil if you're wanting something spicy.

Per Serving: Calories: 202; Total fat: 12g; Saturated fat: 2g; Sodium: 224mg; Total carbohydrates: 19g; Sugar: 4g; Fiber: 5g; Net carbohydrates: 14g; Protein: 7g

Red Lentil Sloppy Joes with Roasted Asparagus

30 MINUTES OR LESS, SOY-FREE, VEGAN

Serves 2
Prep time: 8 minutes

Cook time: 20 minutes

This recipe is a modern take on the American classic with healthier lentils in place of ground beef. You can use sandwich thins or cauliflower thins or serve the tasty filling open-faced; there are countless options to choose from to cut carbs. Keep it to one serving of carbohydrates, 15 grams per serving, if using the bread option, or use lettuce instead.

1 bunch aspar-
agus, woody
ends removed

1 tablespoon
extra-virgin olive
oil, divided

½ cup chopped onion

2 teaspoons chopped
serrano pepper
(optional)

2 garlic cloves, minced

1½ cups water

½ cup red len-
tils, rinsed

2 tablespoons ketchup

1 teaspoon paprika

2 cauliflower sand-
wich thin or other
bread option

1. Preheat the oven to 450°F. Line a baking sheet with parchment paper.
2. In a small bowl, toss the asparagus with 1½ teaspoons of olive oil until well coated, and spread the vegetable on the prepared baking sheet. Bake for 12 to 15 minutes.
3. Meanwhile, in a medium saucepan over medium heat, heat the remaining 1½ teaspoons of olive oil and sauté the onion and serrano pepper (if using) until soft and translucent, 2 to 3 minutes. Add the garlic and cook for 1 minute.
4. Add the water and lentils and bring to a boil. Reduce the heat to low and simmer, stirring occasionally, until the lentils are tender but not falling apart, about 10 minutes.
5. Add the ketchup and paprika. Adjust seasonings as desired and allow the mixture to thicken over the heat for a couple of minutes.
6. Serve on a sandwich thin or slice of bread with a side of roasted asparagus.

Variation:

Serve with an assortment of raw veggies if you prefer to skip the asparagus.

Per Serving: Calories: 352; Total fat: 12g; Saturated fat: 3g; Sodium: 317mg; Total carbohydrates: 45g; Sugar: 8g; Fiber: 10g; Net carbohydrates: 35g; Protein: 20g

First-of-the-Season Tomato, Peach, and Strawberry Salad

30 MINUTES OR LESS, GLUTEN-FREE, NUT-FREE, ONE-POT, SOY-FREE, VEGAN

Serves 6   **Prep time:** 15 minutes

This combination of fruits over greens is beyond refreshing on a spring or summer day. Pairing the sweet, sour, and tangy flavors of in-season ripe tomatoes with peach and strawberry, this lovely salad is balanced out by spring greens. Bursting with nutrients, it's a winning recipe that takes almost no time to prepare.

6 cups mixed spring greens

4 large ripe plum tomatoes, thinly sliced

4 large ripe peaches, pitted and thinly sliced

12 ripe strawberries, thinly sliced

½ Vidalia onion, thinly sliced

2 tablespoons white balsamic vinegar

2 tablespoons extra-virgin olive oil

Freshly ground black pepper

1. Put the greens in a large salad bowl, and layer the tomatoes, peaches, strawberries, and onion on top.
2. Dress with the vinegar and olive oil, toss together, and season with pepper.

Variation:

If you don't have access to peaches or strawberries, use any available stone fruit along with any berry of your choice.

Per Serving (2 cups): Calories: 127; Total fat: 5g; Saturated fat: 0g; Sodium: 30mg; Total carbohydrates: 19g; Sugar: 13g; Fiber: 5g; Net carbohydrates: 14g; Protein: 4g

Grilled Hearts of Romaine with Buttermilk Dressing

30 MINUTES OR LESS, GLUTEN-FREE, NUT-FREE, SOY-FREE, VEGETARIAN

Serves 4
Prep time: 5 minutes

Cook time: 5 minutes

Grilling vegetables that are generally eaten raw gives a chance to experiment with temperature and texture and discover a new taste. As the lettuce cooks, it will soften, and the edges may slightly char. The different textures of the lettuce are a treat, and the zingy dressing is the perfect finishing touch.

For the romaine

2 heads romaine lettuce, halved lengthwise

2 tablespoons extra-virgin olive oil

For the dressing

½ cup low-fat buttermilk

1 tablespoon extra-virgin olive oil

1 garlic clove, pressed

¼ bunch fresh chives, thinly chopped

1 pinch red pepper flakes

To make the romaine

1. Heat a grill pan over medium heat.
2. Brush each lettuce half with some of the olive oil, and place flat-side down on the grill. Grill for 3 to 5 minutes, or until the lettuce slightly wilts and develops light grill marks.

To make the dressing

3. In a small bowl, whisk the buttermilk, 1 tablespoon of the olive oil, garlic, chives, and red pepper flakes together.
4. Drizzle 2 tablespoons of dressing over each romaine half and serve.

Variation:

If you like this dish with a bite, substitute whole radishes for the romaine. Slice the radishes in half, with greens still attached, and follow the same grilling instructions.

Per Serving (½ head): Calories: 126; Total fat: 11g; Saturated fat: 2g; Sodium: 41mg; Total carbohydrates: 12g; Sugar: 5g; Fiber: 7g; Net carbohydrates: 5g; Protein: 5g

Raw Corn Salad with Black-Eyed Peas

30 MINUTES OR LESS, GLUTEN-FREE, NUT-FREE, SOY-FREE, VEGAN

Serves 8   **Prep time:** 15 minutes

Sweet corn is delicious, can be eaten cooked or raw, and tastes excellent either way. Corn has a medium glycemic score of 52, but when combined with other lower-glycemic foods, protein, and fats, the whole meal has a slower release of glucose into the bloodstream. In this fresh salad, the corn's sweetness is tempered by black-eyed peas.

- 2 ears fresh corn, kernels cut off
- 2 cups cooked black-eyed peas
- 1 green bell pepper, seeded and chopped
- ½ red onion, chopped
- 2 celery stalks, finely chopped
- ½ pint cherry tomatoes, halved
- 3 tablespoons white balsamic vinegar
- 2 tablespoons extra-virgin olive oil
- 1 garlic clove, minced
- ¼ teaspoon smoked paprika
- ¼ teaspoon ground cumin
- ¼ teaspoon red pepper flakes

1. In a large salad bowl, combine the corn, black-eyed peas, bell pepper, onion, celery, and tomatoes.
2. In a small bowl, to make the dressing, whisk the vinegar, olive oil, garlic, paprika, cumin, and red pepper flakes together.
3. Pour the dressing over the salad and toss gently to coat. Serve and enjoy.

Prep Tip:

To reduce your preparation time, use frozen or rinsed canned black-eyed peas.

Per Serving (½ cup): Calories: 123; Total fat: 5g; Saturated fat: 1g; Sodium: 24mg; Total carbohydrates: 18g; Sugar: 3g; Fiber: 4g; Net carbohydrates: 14g; Protein: 5g

Chickpea Salad

30 MINUTES OR LESS, NUT-FREE, ONE-POT, GLUTEN-FREE, VEGAN

Serves 4   **Prep time:** 15 minutes

Chickpeas are legumes, which means they are lower in starch than other types of beans but still pack plenty of protein. This recipe features edamame, another legume. Edamame are young soybeans in the pod—but you can buy them shelled and frozen. They have a lovely nutty flavor.

½ cup store-bought balsamic vinaigrette

1 (15-ounce) can chickpeas, drained and rinsed

1 cup cherry tomatoes

1 small red onion, quartered and sliced

2 large cucumbers, peeled and cut into bite-size pieces

1 large zucchini, cut into bite-size pieces

1 (10-ounce) package frozen shelled edamame, steamed or microwaved

Chopped fresh parsley, for garnish

1. Pour the vinaigrette into a large bowl. Add the chickpeas, tomatoes, onion, cucumbers, zucchini, and edamame and toss until all the ingredients are coated

2. Garnish with chopped parsley.

Prep Tip:

You can buy precut zucchini in the produce section of your supermarket or start with frozen to reduce prep time.

Per Serving: Calories: 294; Total fat: 12g; Saturated fat: 2g; Sodium: 298mg; Total carbohydrates: 35g; Sugar: 14g; Fiber: 11g; Net carbohydrates: 24g; Protein: 15g

Easy Chop Salad

30 MINUTES OR LESS, DAIRY-FREE, GLUTEN-FREE, NUT-FREE, ONE-POT, SOY-FREE

Serves 2   **Prep time:** 10 minutes

Chopped salads are fantastic because they are so easy to customize to your taste. Just chop up a bunch of different veggies, add some chopped meat, and toss with dressing, and you've got a tasty meal on the go. This version uses turkey, but you can make it vegetarian by adding hard-boiled egg whites, olives, and additional veggies. Or get creative and add what you have in the refrigerator.

2 cups chopped iceberg lettuce

10 cherry tomatoes, halved

½ cup pitted black olives, chopped

6 ounces turkey, chopped

½ red onion, chopped

1 red bell pepper, seeded and chopped

10 basil leaves, torn

¼ cup Italian Vinaigrette (page 218)

1. In a large bowl, combine the lettuce, tomatoes, olives, turkey, onion, bell pepper, and basil leaves.
2. Toss with the vinaigrette just before serving.

Storage Tip:

The salad will store for up to 3 days in the refrigerator. The vinaigrette will store in the refrigerator for up to a week.

Variation:

You can also balance this chopped salad by adding a vegetarian source of protein and ½ cup of kidney beans, which would add 15 grams of carbs.

Per Serving: Calories: 305; Total fat: 20g; Saturated fat: 3g; Sodium: 1271mg; Total carbohydrates: 17g; Sugar: 10g; Fiber: 5g; Net carbohydrates: 12g; Protein: 18g

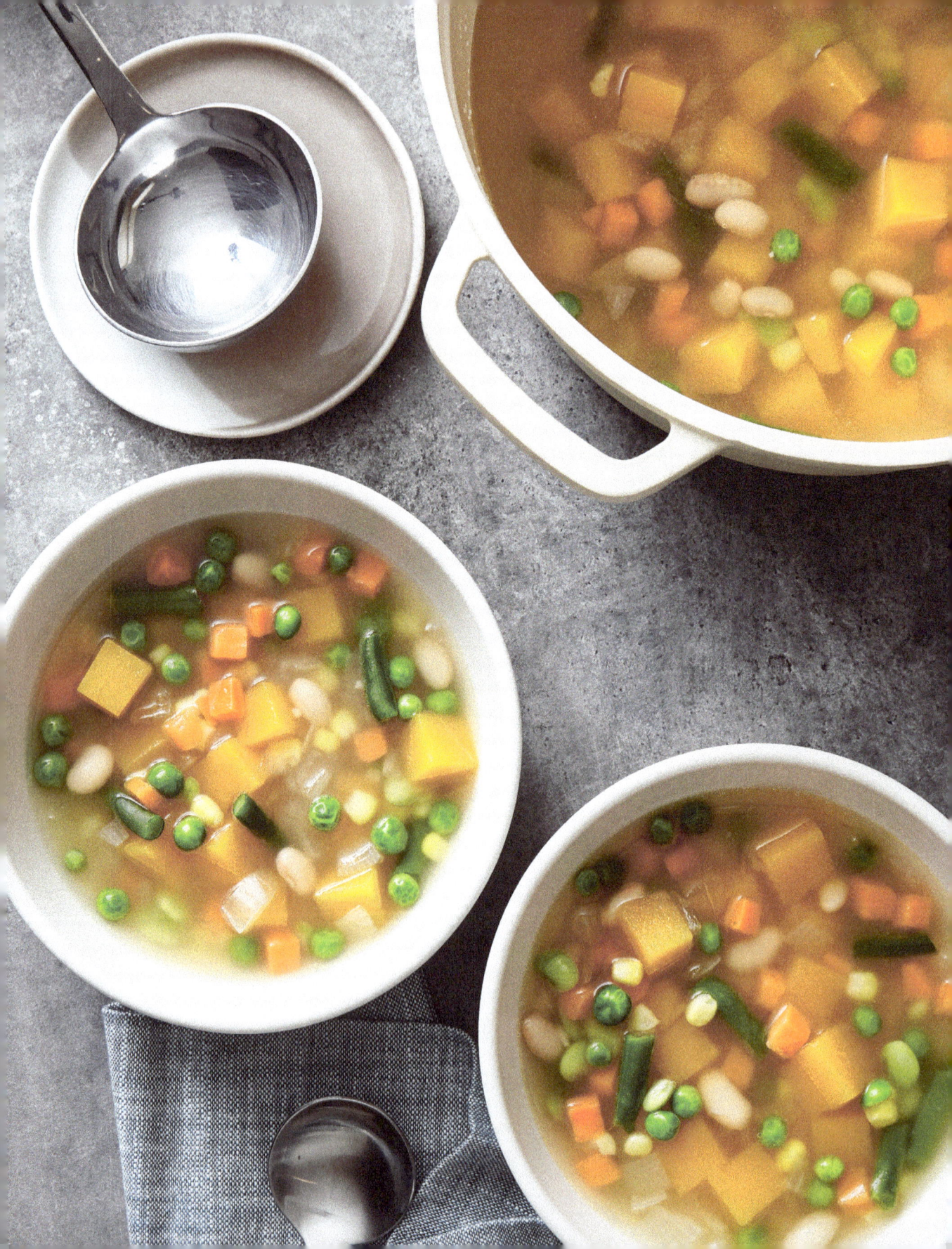

Butternut and Bean Soup

NUT-FREE, ONE-POT, SOY-FREE, VEGAN

Serves 4
Prep time: 10 minutes

Cook time: 35 minutes

A piping-hot bowl of soup is welcome any time of the year, but especially during the winter months. This nutritious and filling recipe takes advantage of peak winter squash season. You can switch up the vegetables depending on what is in your refrigerator, garden, or freezer. The protein in this soup comes from beans, so it's great for vegans!

1 tablespoon avocado oil

1 medium onion, chopped

1 teaspoon minced garlic

1 cup cubed butternut squash

4 cups low-sodium vegetable broth

1 (16-ounce) bag frozen mixed vegetables (no need to thaw)

1 (15-ounce) can great northern beans, drained and rinsed

1 tablespoon salt-free seasoning blend, such as Mrs. Dash, or freshly ground black pepper

1. In a stockpot over medium heat, heat the avocado oil until it shimmers. Add the onion, garlic, and squash and sauté until soft, about 3 minutes.
2. Add the broth, frozen vegetables, beans, and seasoning and stir until combined.
3. Bring the liquid to a boil, then turn the heat to low. Cover and simmer, stirring occasionally, for 30 minutes, or until all the ingredients are tender.

Storage Tip:

Refrigerate leftover soup in an airtight container for up to 5 days or freeze for up to 3 months. Thaw your frozen soup in the refrigerator overnight and reheat in the microwave or a stockpot.

Prep Tip:

You can buy squash already peeled, seeded, and precut in your grocer's produce section, or buy frozen squash chunks.

Per Serving: Calories: 211; Total fat: 4g; Saturated fat: 0g; Sodium: 114mg; Total carbohydrates: 36g; Sugar: 6g; Fiber: 11g; Net carbohydrates: 25g; Protein: 9g

Spicy Corn and Shrimp Salad in Avocado

30 MINUTES OR LESS, DAIRY-FREE, GLUTEN-FREE, NUT-FREE, SOY-FREE

Serves 2   **Prep time:** 10 minutes

An avocado half makes the perfect vehicle for a spicy shrimp, corn, and bell pepper salad. Its creamy texture goes well with the crisp corn and bell peppers, and it's a good source of healthy fats. Plus, the briny shrimp just tastes delicious when combined with earthy corn, sweet bell peppers, and grassy avocados.

¼ cup mayonnaise

1 teaspoon sriracha (or to taste)

½ teaspoon grated lemon zest

¼ teaspoon kosher salt

4 ounces cooked baby shrimp

½ cup canned low-sodium corn kernels

½ red bell pepper, seeded and chopped

1 avocado, halved lengthwise

1. In a medium bowl, combine the mayonnaise, sriracha, lemon zest, and salt.
2. Add the shrimp, corn, and bell pepper. Mix to combine.
3. Spoon the mixture into the avocado halves.

Storage Tip:

The shrimp salad will keep for up to 3 days in the refrigerator. Don't cut the avocado until you're ready to serve.

Variation:

Corn is considered a starch, with similar amounts of carbohydrates as peas or pasta—½ cup of corn has 15 grams of carbs. Depending on your carb needs, add or subtract corn in this easy recipe.

Per Serving: Calories: 320; Total fat: 21g; Saturated fat: 3g; Sodium: 328mg; Total carbohydrates: 21g; Sugar: 4g; Fiber: 8g; Net carbohydrates: 13g; Protein: 17g

Egg Drop Soup

30 MINUTES OR LESS, DAIRY-FREE, NUT-FREE, VEGETARIAN

Serves 4
Prep time: 10 minutes

Cook time: 15 minutes

Egg drop soup has long been a staple of Chinese buffets in the United States. This flavor-packed soup, with its whisper-thin strands of egg and light crunch of scallion, is a favorite for many people. It is a lovely cold-weather dish.

3½ cups low-sodium vegetable broth, divided

1 teaspoon grated fresh ginger (optional)

2 garlic cloves, minced

1 tablespoon reduced-sodium soy sauce or tamari

1 tablespoon cornstarch

2 large eggs, lightly beaten

2 scallions, both white and green parts, thinly sliced

1. In a large saucepan, bring 3 cups plus 6 tablespoons of vegetable broth and the ginger (if using), garlic, and soy sauce to a boil over medium-high heat.
2. In a small bowl, make a slurry by combining the cornstarch and the remaining 2 tablespoons of broth. Stir until dissolved. Slowly add the cornstarch mixture to the rest of the heated soup, stirring until thickened, 2 to 3 minutes.
3. Reduce the heat to low and simmer. While stirring the soup, pour the eggs in slowly.
4. Turn off the heat, add the scallions, and serve.

Storage Tip:

Refrigerate the cooled soup in an airtight container for up to 3 days.

Per Serving: Calories: 66; Total fat: 3g; Saturated fat: 1g; Sodium: 165mg; Total carbohydrates: 6g; Sugar: 0g; Fiber: 1g; Net carbohydrates: 5g; Protein: 4g

Lemony Chicken Noodle Soup

DAIRY-FREE, NUT-FREE, ONE-POT, SOY-FREE

Serves 4

Prep time: 15 minutes

Cook time: 25 minutes

The whole family will love this belly-warming soup so much that you might want to make a double or triple batch to freeze for when life gets busy. It balances fresh vegetables and seasonings with lean protein, and the lemon provides a little kick.

1 pound boneless, skinless chicken breast, cut into ½-inch strips

⅔ cup sliced leek

1 teaspoon dried dill

¼ teaspoon freshly ground black pepper

4 cups low-sodium chicken broth

1 tablespoon freshly squeezed lemon juice

1 cup uncooked no-yolk wide egg noodles

1 (9-ounce) package frozen green beans (no need to thaw)

1. In a stockpot, combine the chicken, leek, dill, pepper, broth, and lemon juice.
2. Bring to a boil over high heat, then reduce the heat to medium. Cook for 10 minutes, stirring once during the cooking time.
3. Add the egg noodles and green beans and simmer for about 15 minutes, until the noodles are tender.

Prep Tip:

When buying fresh leeks, look for smaller, more flavorful stalks that are firm and light green. If you can't find leeks, substitute sliced scallions.

Per Serving: Calories: 197; Total fat: 3g; Saturated fat: 0g; Sodium: 143mg; Total carbohydrates: 14g; Sugar: 2g; Fiber: 3g; Net carbohydrates: 11g; Protein: 28g

Turkey Chili

NUT-FREE, ONE-POT, SOY-FREE

Serves 4
Prep time: 10 minutes

Cook time: 25 minutes

This chili recipe works for a busy weeknight dinner or for the big game! You can make it as hot or mild as you like by adjusting the chili powder or adding a dash of hot sauce at the end. Be sure to buy the leanest ground turkey you can find, or ask the butcher to grind lean turkey breast for you.

1 pound extra-lean ground turkey

1 large onion, chopped

2 (28-ounce) cans reduced-sodium diced tomatoes

1 (15-ounce) can red kidney beans, drained and rinsed

1 (4½-ounce) can chopped green chiles, drained

¼ cup salsa

2 teaspoons chili powder

1. In a stockpot, brown the ground turkey and onion over medium heat, about 5 minutes, breaking up the meat with a wooden spoon as it cooks.
2. Add the tomatoes with their juices, beans, chiles, and salsa and mix well. Stir in the chili powder.
3. Lower the heat and cook for about 20 minutes, until warmed through and the flavors blend.
4. Divide the soup into 4 bowls and serve.

Storage Tip:

This is a great recipe to double up or adjust as needed when feeding a crowd. Refrigerate the chili in an airtight container for up to 4 days or freeze for up to 3 months. Thaw in the refrigerator overnight and reheat in the microwave or a stockpot.

Per Serving: Calories: 339; Total fat: 11g; Saturated fat: 3g; Sodium: 287mg; Total carbohydrates: 33g; Sugar: 12g; Fiber: 15g; Net carbohydrates: 18g; Protein: 32g

Spicy Vegetarian Chili

30 MINUTES OR LESS, GLUTEN-FREE, NUT-FREE, ONE-POT, SOY-FREE, VEGAN

Serves 6

Prep time: 5 minutes

Cook time: 15 minutes

This meatless meal is a spicy addition to your weekday routine. It takes very little prep, and because most of the ingredients are canned, you can keep them in your pantry and be ready to cook at any time. To keep things super easy, empty all the beans into a colander, then rinse and drain them together.

- 1 (15-ounce) can chickpeas, drained and rinsed
- 1 (15-ounce) can black beans, drained and rinsed
- 1 (15-ounce) can whole-kernel corn (or frozen corn), drained
- 1 (28-ounce) can reduced-sodium diced tomatoes
- 1 (4-ounce) can chopped green chiles, drained
- 1 large onion, chopped
- 1 large green bell pepper, seeded and chopped
- ½ teaspoon ground cumin
- ½ teaspoon chili powder
- ¼ cup guacamole (optional)

1. In a Dutch oven, combine the chickpeas, beans, corn, tomatoes with their juices, chiles, onion, bell pepper, cumin, and chili powder. Heat over medium heat, stirring occasionally, until the mixture is heated through, about 15 minutes.
2. Top each serving with 1 tablespoon of guacamole, if desired.

Variation:

You can include vegetarian beef crumbles to add texture and body to this recipe while keeping it vegan. If you like it spicy, add a chopped jalapeño pepper to the pot.

Per Serving: Calories: 202; Total fat: 3g; Saturated fat: 0g; Sodium: 269mg; Total carbohydrates: 39g; Sugar: 8g; Fiber: 12g; Net carbohydrates: 27g; Protein: 10g

Chickpea, Tomato, and Kale Soup

30 MINUTES OR LESS, GLUTEN-FREE, NUT-FREE, ONE-POT, SOY-FREE, VEGAN

Serves 4
Prep time: 10 minutes

Cook time: 15 minutes

Nothing sounds quite so good on a brisk day as a delicious bowl of hot soup. Using ingredients that come together easily, this hearty soup overflows with fiber, vitamins A and C, and potassium. Be sure to use low-sodium varieties when buying canned goods. This soup is perfect for a quick dinner solution—just 10 minutes of prep and 15 minutes to cook.

1 tablespoon extra-virgin olive oil

1 onion, chopped

3 garlic cloves, minced

1 (15-ounce) can low-sodium chickpeas, drained and rinsed

1 (15-ounce) can no-salt-added diced tomatoes

4 cups low-sodium vegetable broth

4 cups finely chopped kale leaves

½ teaspoon kosher salt

Freshly ground black pepper

1. In a large pot over medium-high heat, heat the olive oil. Add the onion and garlic and sauté for 3 to 5 minutes, until softened.
2. Stir in the chickpeas and tomatoes with their juices. Add the vegetable broth and bring to a boil. Reduce the heat to low, add the kale, and simmer for 2 to 3 minutes, until the kale wilts. Season with the salt and pepper. Serve.

Prep Tip:

Save time on chopping by purchasing a bag of prechopped kale. Alternatively, baby kale leaves are also a quick option that requires no prep work. The tender leaves cook more quickly than mature ones, so cut the simmer time to 1 minute.

Per Serving: Calories: 146; Total fat: 6g; Saturated fat: 1g; Sodium: 284mg; Total carbohydrates: 21g; Sugar: 6g; Fiber: 7g; Net carbohydrates: 14g; Protein: 5g

Tomato-Basil Soup with Grilled Cheese Croutons

30 MINUTES OR LESS, NUT-FREE, SOY-FREE, VEGETARIAN

Serves 4

Prep time: 10 minutes

Cook time: 20 minutes

Tomato soup does not have to be the pale, bland canned version; it can be vibrant and bursting with summer flavor and bright color. Fresh tomatoes are ideal for this recipe when they're in season during the summer and autumn, but there's nothing wrong with canned. Outside of this harvest time frame, fresh tomatoes tend to be mealy and mushy.

For the tomato soup

- 2 tablespoons extra-virgin olive oil
- 1 onion, chopped
- 1 tablespoon minced garlic
- 3 pounds fresh tomatoes, cored and chopped, or canned diced tomatoes
- 8 cups low-sodium vegetable broth
- ¼ cup tomato paste
- ½ cup low-fat Greek yogurt
- ½ teaspoon garlic powder
- Pinch kosher salt
- Pinch freshly ground black pepper
- ⅓ cup fresh basil, chopped

For the grilled cheese croutons

- Nonstick cooking spray
- 4 slices whole wheat bread
- 2 ounces cheese (cheddar or Gruyère), shredded
- Freshly ground black pepper (optional)

To make the tomato soup

1. In a medium stockpot over medium heat, heat the olive oil. Sauté the onion and minced garlic until translucent, about 3 minutes.
2. Add the tomatoes and vegetable broth, increase the heat to medium-high, cover, and simmer until the tomato skin wrinkles and pulls back from the tomato flesh, 8 to 10 minutes.
3. Add the tomato paste, yogurt, garlic powder, salt, and pepper and simmer for 3 to 5 minutes.
4. Transfer the soup to a blender and blend until smooth, in batches if necessary. Leave the center piece out of the lid and cover the lid with a clean kitchen towel while blending to allow the steam to escape.
5. Serve the soup topped with basil and the grilled cheese croutons (if using).

To make the grilled cheese croutons

6. Spray one side of each slice of bread with nonstick cooking spray.
7. Put a small nonstick skillet over medium heat, and place 1 slice of bread in the skillet, buttered-side down. Top with half of the cheese and season with pepper (if using). Then top with the second slice of bread, buttered-side up. When the underside is golden brown, 3 to 4 minutes, turn the sandwich. Cook until the second side of the bread is golden and crispy.
8. Repeat with the remaining ingredients.
9. Cut each sandwich into 1-inch squares and use them to garnish the soup.

Storage Tip:

Refrigerate the cooled soup in an airtight container for 3 to 5 days. Keep the garnishes separate.

Variation:

If you want to cut down on carbohydrates but still want the grilled cheese, use half the bread, cube it into ¼-inch-square pieces, and brown them in a skillet with 1 teaspoon of olive oil or fat. Sprinkle the cubes on the tomato soup followed by the shredded cheese.

Per Serving: Calories: 304; Total fat: 13g; Saturated fat: 3g; Sodium: 244mg; Total carbohydrates: 37g; Sugar: 16g; Fiber: 7g; Net carbohydrates: 30g; Protein: 14g

Lentil and Vegetable Soup

GLUTEN-FREE, NUT-FREE, ONE-POT, SOY-FREE, VEGAN

Serves 6
Prep time: 10 minutes

Cook time: 30 minutes

Lentils are one of the most versatile and nutritious foods for regulating blood sugar. They are low in fat, cholesterol-free, high in folate, potassium, and iron, and a rich source of fiber. Combined with vegetables, it's a nutritional match made in heaven. Best of all, unlike other legumes, lentils require no presoaking, making them perfect for a weeknight meal. Make life simple and healthier—start eating lentils today!

- 2 tablespoons extra-virgin olive oil
- 2 carrots, chopped
- 2 celery stalks, chopped
- 1 onion, chopped
- 3 garlic cloves, minced
- 2 cups dried brown lentils, rinsed
- 4 cups low-sodium vegetable broth
- 1 cup water
- 4 cups chopped fresh spinach
- ½ teaspoon kosher salt
- ¼ teaspoon freshly ground black pepper

1. In a large pot over medium heat, heat the olive oil. Add the carrots, celery, onion, and garlic, and sauté for 3 to 5 minutes, until the onion is softened.
2. Add the lentils, vegetable broth, and water, and bring to a boil. Reduce the heat to low, cover, and simmer for 20 minutes, until the lentils are tender.
3. Turn off the heat and stir in the spinach. Let stand for 1 to 2 minutes, until the greens are wilted.
4. Season with the salt and pepper and serve.

Variation:

Vegetable broth gives this soup a lovely flavor, while keeping it vegetarian. However, feel free to use chicken broth or even water to make this soup. If you do use water, add a bit more salt and be sure to taste it before serving.

Per Serving: Calories: 290; Total fat: 5g; Saturated fat: 1g; Sodium: 165mg; Total carbohydrates: 44g; Sugar: 2g; Fiber: 9g; Net carbohydrates: 33g; Protein: 17g

Black Bean Soup

30 MINUTES OR LESS, GLUTEN-FREE, NUT-FREE, ONE-POT, SOY-FREE, VEGAN

Serves 4
Prep time: 5 minutes

Cook time: 20 minutes

Talk about a flavorful soup! Simple to put together and ready in less than 30 minutes, this is a recipe you'll come back to often. Black beans are a powerhouse of protein, fiber, magnesium, potassium, and vitamin K, and this recipe makes one of the most satisfying, hearty soups—good any time of year. Throw in some frozen corn or fire-roasted tomatoes to ramp up the flavor if you like. Pair it with a dark leafy green salad, and you've got a meal to feel good about.

2 tablespoons
extra-virgin olive oil

1 onion, chopped

3 garlic cloves, minced

2 (15-ounce) cans
black beans, drained
and rinsed

3 cups low-sodium
vegetable broth

1 teaspoon
ground cumin

½ teaspoon kosher salt

1. In a large pot over medium-high heat, heat the olive oil. Add the onion and garlic, and sauté for 3 to 5 minutes, until softened.
2. Stir in the black beans, vegetable broth, cumin, and salt. Bring to a boil, reduce the heat to maintain a simmer, and cook for 10 minutes, until slightly thickened and the flavors meld.
3. Using a potato masher, mash about half the beans in the soup and serve.

Storage Tip:

Soups tend to get better with age as the flavors meld. This soup will keep well for about 4 days in the refrigerator, so make it early in the week and enjoy it when you need a quick meal.

Per Serving: Calories: 246; Total fat: 8g; Saturated fat: 1g; Sodium: 248mg; Total carbohydrates: 34g; Sugar: 1g; Fiber: 12g; Net carbohydrates: 22g; Protein: 12g

Falafel Sandwich

30 MINUTES OR LESS, NUT-FREE, SOY-FREE, VEGETARIAN

Serves 6
Prep time: 15 minutes

Cook time: 15 minutes

Falafel is one of the most delicious ways to get more chickpeas on the menu. Nestled in pita bread (use whole wheat bread for added nutrition), these Middle Eastern chickpea patties, seasoned with onion and spices, make a filling legume-based meal. You can also skip the pitas, serving the falafel on a bed of lightly seasoned greens.

2 (15-ounce) cans chickpeas, drained and rinsed

1 medium onion, coarsely chopped

5 garlic cloves, minced, divided

¼ cup packed fresh parsley leaves

Juice of 1 lemon

2 tablespoons extra-virgin olive oil, divided

1 teaspoon ground cumin

1 teaspoon ground coriander

1¼ teaspoons kosher salt, divided

2 teaspoons baking powder

6 large lettuce leaves

Sliced cucumbers, for serving

Sliced tomatoes, for serving

½ cup plain nonfat Greek yogurt

1. In a food processor, combine the chickpeas, onion, 3 garlic cloves, parsley, lemon juice, 1 tablespoon of olive oil, cumin, coriander, and 1 teaspoon of salt. Pulse several times, until the chickpeas and onions are chopped coarsely and mixed but not pureed. Add the baking powder and pulse several more times, until it is mixed in and the mixture forms into a ball. Form the mixture into 12 small balls and press the balls into patties.
2. In a small bowl, whisk the yogurt with the remaining ¼ teaspoon of salt and 2 garlic cloves. Set aside.
3. In a large skillet over medium heat, heat the remaining 1 tablespoon of olive oil.
4. Working in batches, cook the patties for 2 to 3 minutes per side, gently flipping once during cooking, until browned and crisp.
5. To serve, place two patties into a lettuce leaf, top with cucumber and tomato slices, and garnish with a spoonful of yogurt.

Per Serving: Calories: 206; Total fat: 7g; Saturated fat: 1g; Sodium: 428mg; Total carbohydrates: 27g; Sugar: 6g; Fiber: 7g; Net carbohydrates: 20g; Protein: 10g

Simple Salmon Burgers

30 MINUTES OR LESS, DAIRY-FREE, NUT-FREE, SOY-FREE

Serves 4
Prep time: 10 minutes

Cook time: 10 minutes

For a nutritious and tasty twist, replace ground beef with heart-healthy, omega-3-rich salmon. These easy salmon burgers make for a light dinner you can have ready in under 30 minutes on busy weeknights. To save on carbs, skip the bun and serve the patties over a bed of salad greens lightly seasoned with vinegar and oil.

2 (6-ounce) cans boneless, skinless salmon

1 large egg

½ cup whole wheat bread crumbs

2 garlic cloves, minced

Juice of 1 lemon

1 tablespoon whole-grain or Dijon mustard

¼ teaspoon kosher salt

¼ teaspoon freshly ground black pepper

1 tablespoon extra-virgin olive oil

4 whole wheat hamburger buns

Lettuce, for serving

Sliced tomato, for serving

Mayonnaise, for serving

1. In a large bowl, stir together the salmon, egg, bread crumbs, garlic, lemon juice, mustard, salt, and pepper. Form the mixture into 4 patties.
2. In a large skillet over medium-high heat, heat the olive oil.
3. Add the patties and cook for 4 to 5 minutes per side, until golden brown.
4. Serve on the buns, topped with lettuce, tomato, and mayonnaise.

Prep Tip:

Prepare the burgers the night before and refrigerate until ready to cook.

Per Serving: Calories: 325; Total fat: 11g; Saturated fat: 2g; Sodium: 492mg; Total carbohydrates: 34g; Sugar: 6g; Fiber: 5g; Net carbohydrates: 29g; Protein: 24g

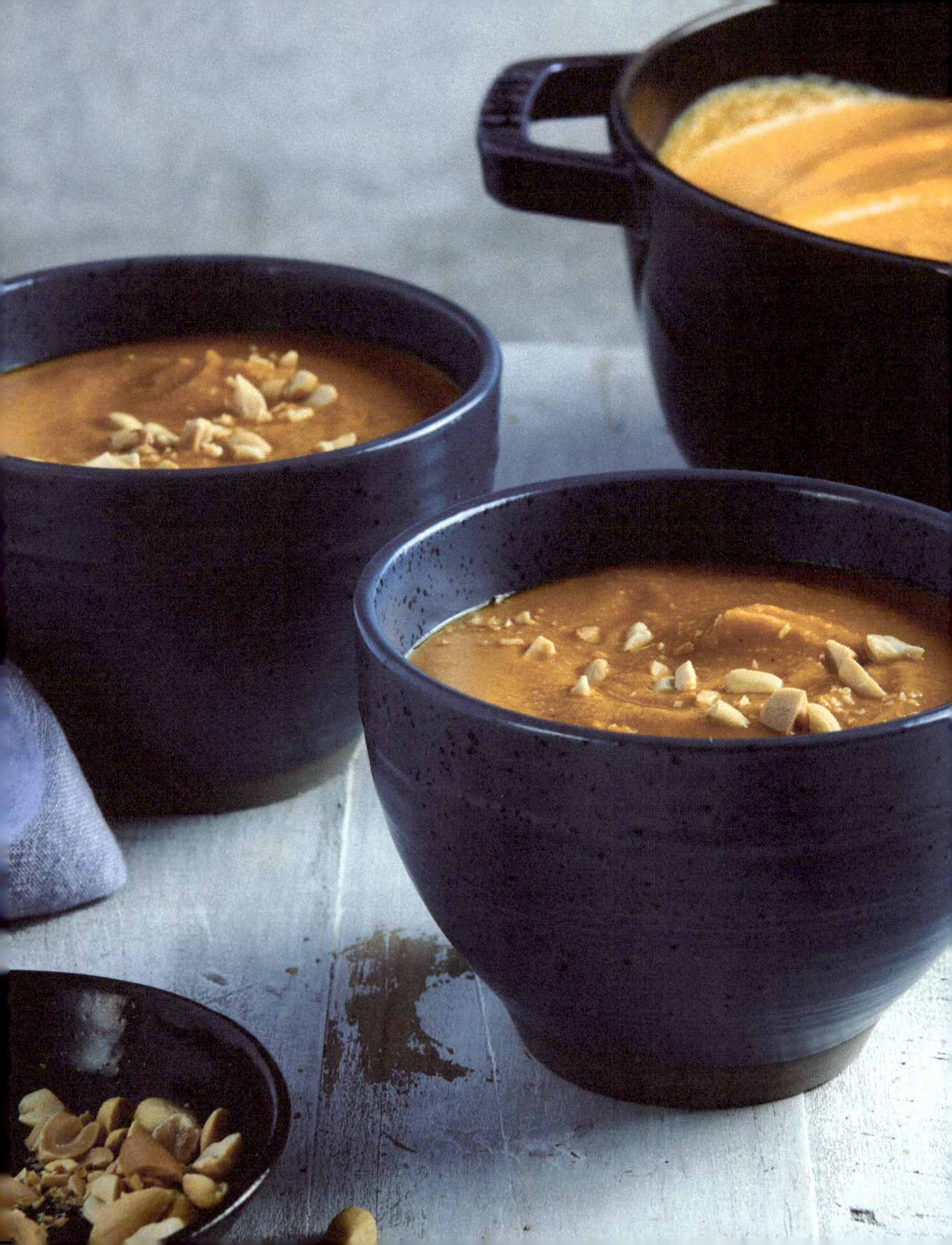

Sweet Potato and Pumpkin Soup with Peanuts

GLUTEN-FREE, SOY-FREE, VEGAN

Serves 8
Prep time: 10 minutes

Cook time: 45 minutes

A Southern take on a West African peanut soup, this soup has a savory yet still sweet and nutty flavor. Peanuts are a great source of heart-healthy fats and plant-based protein. This dish calls for fresh pumpkin, but you can use additive-free canned pumpkin for a similar taste.

3 cups Vegetable Broth (page 225) or store-bought low-sodium vegetable broth, divided

1 celery stalk, coarsely chopped

1 cup coarsely chopped tomato

1 red bell pepper, seeded and chopped

1 large sweet potato, peeled and cut into 2-inch cubes

1 small pumpkin, peeled and cut into 2-inch cubes

1 bay leaf

1 teaspoon paprika

2 cups roasted unsalted peanuts

Baby sage leaves (optional)

1. In a large Dutch oven, bring 1 cup of broth to a simmer over medium heat.
2. Add the celery, tomato, and bell pepper and cook for 5 to 7 minutes, or until softened.
3. Add the sweet potato, pumpkin, bay leaf, paprika, and the remaining 2 cups of broth. Cover and cook for 30 minutes, or until the sweet potato and pumpkin are soft.
4. Add the peanuts and cook for 5 minutes, or until the peanuts become less crunchy. Discard the bay leaf.
5. Transfer to a heat-safe blender, and pulse until the soup has a batter-like consistency.

Prep Tip:

If you prefer a less-nutty flavor, reduce the quantity of peanuts, or simply use ½ cup as garnish and divide it between each serving.

Per Serving (¾ cup): Calories: 266; Total fat: 18g; Saturated fat: 3g; Sodium: 50mg; Total carbohydrates: 19g; Sugar: 6g; Fiber: 5g; Net carbohydrates: 14g; Protein: 12g

Greek Salad with Feta and Olives

30 MINUTES OR LESS, GLUTEN-FREE, NUT-FREE, ONE-POT, SOY-FREE, VEGETARIAN

Serves 4   **Prep time:** 15 minutes

Greek salad is like a flavor explosion. From the buttery olives to the grassy bite of feta to the fragrant herbs in the vinaigrette, it's a tasty salad that tends to be low in carbohydrates. Add whole-grain bread sticks, pita, or stuffed grape leaves if you want to add more carbs. Count the added rice in the grape leaves. To keep salad crisp, mix in the dressing just before serving.

4 cups chopped iceberg lettuce

1 cucumber, chopped

10 cherry tomatoes, halved

½ cup pitted black olives

¼ cup crumbled feta cheese

½ red onion, thinly sliced

½ cup Greek Vinaigrette (page 218)

1. In a large bowl, combine the lettuce, cucumber, tomatoes, olives, feta, and onion. Toss to combine.
2. Toss with the dressing just before serving.

Storage Tip:

This salad will store for up to 3 days in the refrigerator. The vinaigrette will store in the refrigerator for up to a week.

Variation:

Add some whole wheat croutons for crunch and to boost carbs; ¼ cup of whole wheat croutons adds 15 grams of carbs.

Per Serving: Calories: 199; Total fat: 17g; Saturated fat: 3g; Sodium: 299mg; Total carbohydrates: 9g; Sugar: 4g; Fiber: 3g; Net carbohydrates: 6g; Protein: 3g

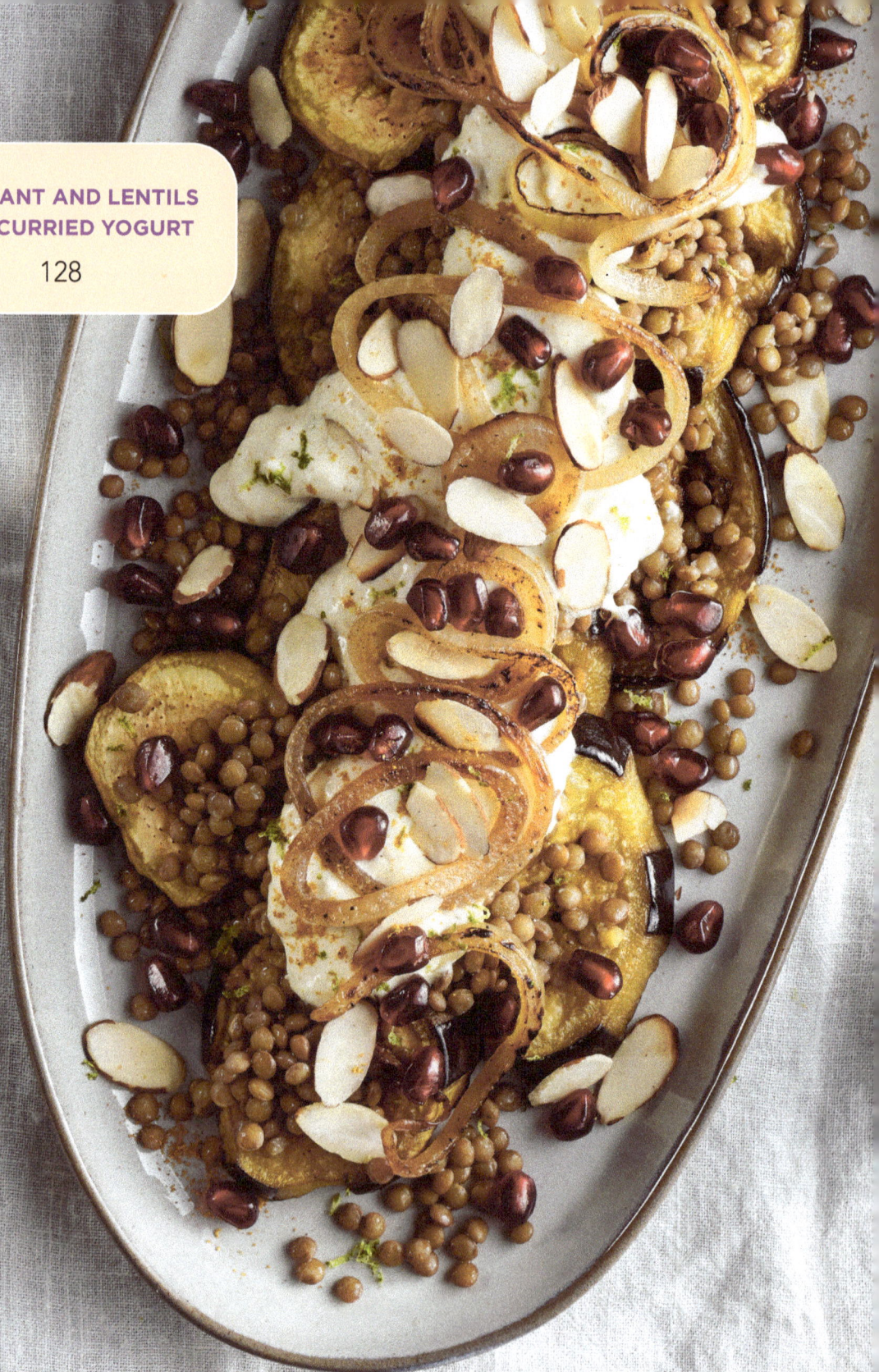

**EGGPLANT AND LENTILS
WITH CURRIED YOGURT**

128

5

VEGETARIAN MAINS

Bulgur, Lentil, and Spinach Pilaf

NUT-FREE, ONE-POT, SOY-FREE, VEGAN

Serves 4
Prep time: 10 minutes

Cook time: 45 minutes

Pilaf is a dish in which rice or another grain is cooked in a stock. The grains come out separate and fluffy and flavorful. This recipe uses whole-grain wheat bulgur, which is the berry of wheat grain, as well as lentils. The bulgur and lentil are inexpensive proteins, which make this a meatless, low-fat, budget-friendly meal.

1 tablespoon
extra-virgin olive oil

½ cup
uncooked bulgur

1 medium
onion, chopped

2 cups low-sodium
vegetable broth

1 (15-ounce) can
lentils, rinsed
and drained

1 (12-ounce) package
frozen chopped
spinach, thawed and
well drained

½ teaspoon freshly
ground black pepper

1. In a large stockpot, heat the olive oil over medium heat. Add the bulgur and sauté until toasted, about 5 minutes. Add the onion and cook until soft, about 5 minutes.
2. Add the broth, cover, and cook for 15 minutes.
3. Remove the pot from the heat and let stand, covered, for 10 to 15 minutes to allow the bulgur to absorb the liquid. Fluff the bulgur with a fork.
4. Add the lentils, spinach, and pepper. Warm over low heat until the spinach and lentils are heated through, about 5 minutes.

Prep Tip:

Don't use finely ground bulgur wheat; because of its short cooking time, it may end up sticking together in a clump. Medium or coarse varieties work best in soups and stews.

Per Serving: Calories: 216; Total fat: 4g; Saturated fat: 0g; Sodium: 108mg; Total carbohydrates: 35g; Sugar: 3g; Fiber: 12g; Net carbohydrates: 23g; Protein: 13g

Summer Squash Casserole

NUT-FREE, SOY-FREE, VEGETARIAN

Serves 8
Prep time: 15 minutes

Cook time: 30 minutes

If you live somewhere with access to a garden plot, summer squash deserves a spot on your planting list thanks to its abundant yield and delicious flavor. Even if you don't have a garden, you can enjoy this hearty casserole during the warmer months, when summer squash is beyond plentiful.

- 1 tablespoon extra-virgin olive oil
- 6 yellow summer squash, thinly sliced
- 1 large portobello mushroom, thinly sliced
- 1 Vidalia onion, thinly sliced
- 1 cup shredded Parmesan cheese, divided
- ½ cup shredded reduced-fat Swiss cheese or mozzarella
- ½ cup whole wheat bread crumbs
- ½ cup tricolor quinoa
- 1 tablespoon Creole seasoning (see tip, page 176)

1. Preheat the oven to 350°F.
2. In a large cast-iron skillet, heat the olive oil over medium heat.
3. Add the squash, mushroom, and onion, and sauté for 7 to 10 minutes, or until softened.
4. Remove from the heat. Add ½ cup of Parmesan cheese and the Swiss cheese and mix well.
5. In a small bowl, whisk the bread crumbs, quinoa, the remaining ½ cup of Parmesan, and the Creole seasoning together. Evenly distribute over the casserole.
6. Transfer the pan to the oven, and bake for 20 minutes, or until browned. Serve warm and enjoy.

Variation:

If you want to make this casserole gluten-free, swap out the bread crumbs for chickpea crumbs, or increase the amount of quinoa to 1 cup.

Per Serving (½ cup): Calories: 179; Total fat: 8g; Saturated fat: 3g; Sodium: 254mg; Total carbohydrates: 18g; Sugar: 4g; Fiber: 3g; Net carbohydrates: 15g; Protein: 10g

Beet Greens and Black Beans

30 MINUTES OR LESS, GLUTEN-FREE, NUT-FREE, SOY-FREE, VEGAN

Serves 4
Prep time: 10 minutes

Cook time: 20 minutes

Beet tops have a sweet grassy taste and are a fantastic source of polyphenols, which have long been researched for their role in reducing the risk of heart disease. This dish combines black beans, beet greens, and dandelion greens, making a wonderful mix of vitamins, minerals, plant-based proteins, and fiber in one satisfying side.

- 1 tablespoon unsalted non-hydrogenated plant-based butter
- ½ Vidalia onion, thinly sliced
- ½ cup Vegetable Broth (page 225) or store-bought low-sodium vegetable broth
- 1 bunch beet greens, cut into ribbons
- 1 bunch dandelion greens, cut into ribbons
- 1 (15-ounce) can no-salt-added black beans
- Freshly ground black pepper

1. In a medium skillet, melt the butter over low heat. Add the onion and sauté for 3 to 5 minutes, or until the onion is translucent.
2. Add the vegetable broth and greens. Cover the skillet and cook for 7 to 10 minutes, or until the greens are wilted.
3. Add the black beans and cook for 3 to 5 minutes, or until the beans are tender. Season with black pepper.

Variation:

You can swap in a dark leafy green of your choice, such as Swiss chard, collard greens, spinach, or arugula.

Per Serving (1 cup): Calories: 161; Total fat: 4g; Saturated fat: 1g; Sodium: 224mg; Total carbohydrates: 25g; Sugar: 1g; Fiber: 10g; Net carbohydrates: 15g; Protein: 9g

Veggie Frittata

30 MINUTES OR LESS, DAIRY-FREE, NUT-FREE, ONE-POT, SOY-FREE, VEGETARIAN

Serves 4
Prep time: 10 minutes

Cook time: 15 minutes

Frittatas are egg dishes, usually cooked in a skillet and browned on the bottom. Just like omelets, frittatas work with tons of different add-ins, including vegetables, cheese, and meat. Serve this dish for breakfast, or with a simple side salad for lunch or dinner.

4 large eggs

¼ cup low-sodium tomato juice

½ teaspoon freshly ground black pepper or salt-free seasoning blend, such as Mrs. Dash

1 cup chopped broccoli florets

¼ cup diced onion

1 (4-ounce) can sliced mushrooms, well drained

Chopped fresh parsley, for garnish

1. In a nonstick skillet (or a regular skillet sprayed with nonstick cooking spray), combine the eggs, tomato juice, and pepper and beat well. Add the broccoli, onion, and mushrooms and stir to combine.
2. Put the skillet over medium heat and cook the eggs without stirring until they are almost set, 8 to 10 minutes.
3. Remove the skillet from the heat, cover, and let stand for another 5 to 10 minutes, until no liquid egg remains.
4. Garnish with chopped parsley.

Variation:

Because a frittata is so versatile, you can add any ingredients to your egg mixture, based on what you have on hand and what your family prefers. Stick to non-starchy vegetables such as asparagus, green beans, or green peppers. You can also add shredded cheese, diced ham, shredded chicken, or chopped bacon.

Per Serving: Calories: 92; Total fat: 5g; Saturated fat: 2g; Sodium: 89mg; Total carbohydrates: 4g; Sugar: 2g; Fiber: 1g; Net carbohydrates: 3g; Protein: 8g

Butternut Squash and Mushroom Lasagna

NUT-FREE, SOY-FREE, VEGETARIAN

Serves 8

Prep time: 20 minutes, plus 10 minutes to stand

Cook time: 55 minutes

Vegetarian lasagna never tasted so good. Layers of noodles (to shorten cooking time, use the no-boil kind), squash, fresh mushrooms, low-fat cottage cheese, and ricotta cheese combine in this wonderful, warm, and satisfying dish. This meatless meal gets a hearty flavor boost from the mushrooms, while fresh herbs provide a nice flavor punch. Freeze leftovers for a fantastic no-prep meal down the road on a busier day.

1 (2-pound) butternut squash

1 tablespoon extra-virgin olive oil

1 onion, chopped

8 ounces brown mushrooms, chopped

Kosher salt

Freshly ground black pepper

1 (15-ounce) container nonfat cottage cheese

1 cup low-fat ricotta cheese

2 large eggs

3 tablespoons chopped fresh thyme, divided

3 tablespoons chopped fresh sage, divided

1 (9-ounce) package no-boil lasagna noodles

½ cup grated low-fat mozzarella cheese

¼ cup grated Parmesan cheese

1. Poke the squash several times with a fork. Microwave it at high power for 6 to 8 minutes, depending on your microwave, until tender. Set aside and let cool.
2. Preheat the oven to 350°F.
3. Meanwhile, in a large skillet over medium-high heat, heat the olive oil and sauté the onion for 3 to 5 minutes, until softened.
4. Add the mushrooms and cook until the liquid evaporates, about 5 minutes. Season lightly with salt and pepper.
5. In a large bowl, stir together the cottage cheese, ricotta, eggs, and 1½ tablespoons each of thyme and sage until well mixed.
6. Using a vegetable peeler or sharp knife, peel the squash and chop into ½-inch pieces. Transfer to another large bowl, and gently toss with the remaining 1½ tablespoons each of sage and thyme.
7. Spread about 1 cup of the ricotta cheese mixture on the bottom of a 9-by-13-inch baking dish.

8.   Arrange 3 noodles on top of the cheese. On the noodles, spread about 1 cup of the ricotta mixture, 1 cup of the squash, and ½ cup of the mushrooms. Add 3 more noodles and repeat the same process for another layer.
9.   Top with the remaining 3 noodles, the remaining 1 cup of ricotta mixture, the mozzarella, and the Parmesan. Cover the dish with aluminum foil and bake for 40 minutes, until the noodles are softened, and the lasagna is bubbly.
10.   Remove the foil and bake for 5 minutes more, until the top is golden brown. Let stand for 10 minutes before serving.

Per Serving: Calories: 309; Total fat: 8g; Saturated fat: 3g; Sodium: 490mg; Total carbohydrates: 40g; Sugar: 5g; Fiber: 3g; Net carbohydrates: 37g; Protein: 19g

Zoodles with Pea Pesto

30 MINUTES OR LESS, GLUTEN-FREE, SOY-FREE, VEGETARIAN

Serves 2
Prep time: 10 minutes

Cook time: 10 minutes

Peas are a starchy vegetable but can easily fit into a healthy plan. This recipe works best with fresh peas, which have enough texture to hold up in pesto. You can also use shelled edamame in place of the peas here for additional protein and a slightly less-sweet flavor profile.

3 zucchini	2 tablespoons extra-virgin olive oil	Pinch kosher salt	¼ to ½ cup Pea Pesto (page 217)

1. Using a vegetable peeler, cut the zucchini lengthwise into long strips. Use a knife to cut the strips into the desired width. Alternatively, use a spiralizer to cut the zucchini into noodles.
2. In a large skillet over medium-high heat, heat the olive oil until it shimmers. Add the zucchini and cook until it starts to soften, about 3 minutes. Add the salt.
3. Toss the zucchini noodles with the pesto.

Storage Tip:

Both the zucchini noodles and the pesto are best served right away.

Variation:

Butternut squash also makes great noodles, and it's slightly higher in carbs. You can replace the zucchini noodles with butternut noodles (1 cup per serving), which have 16 grams of carbs and 3 grams of fiber per cup.

Per Serving: Calories: 470; Total fat: 36g; Saturated fat: 4g; Sodium: 450mg; Total carbohydrates: 14g; Sugar: 8g; Fiber: 4g; Net carbohydrates: 10g; Protein: 10g

Butternut Noodles with Mushroom Sauce

30 MINUTES OR LESS, GLUTEN-FREE, NUT-FREE, ONE-POT, SOY-FREE, VEGAN

Serves 4
Prep time: 10 minutes

Cook time: 20 minutes

Here's an excellent alternative to a high-carb pasta meal. One butternut squash makes about 3 cups of noodles, so you'll need about a squash and a half for this recipe. You can use a spiralizer, buy the noodles precut in the produce section of the grocery store, or use a vegetable peeler and knife to cut the noodles. One cup of cooked butternut squash is estimated at 16 grams of carbohydrates and is a good source of fiber.

- 2 tablespoons extra-virgin olive oil
- 1 pound cremini mushrooms, sliced
- ½ red onion, finely chopped
- 1 teaspoon dried thyme
- ½ teaspoon kosher salt
- 3 garlic cloves, minced
- ½ cup dry white wine
- Pinch red pepper flakes
- 4 cups butternut noodles

1. In a large skillet over medium-high heat, heat the olive oil until it shimmers. Add the mushrooms, onion, thyme, and salt. Cook, stirring occasionally, until the mushrooms start to brown, about 6 minutes. Add the garlic and cook, stirring constantly, for 30 seconds. Add the white wine and red pepper flakes. Stir to combine.
2. Add the noodles. Cook, stirring occasionally, until the noodles are tender, about 5 minutes, and serve.

Storage Tip:

Veggie noodles don't keep well once they're cooked, so it's best to make them fresh. You can make the sauce ahead, store that in the refrigerator for up to 3 days, reheat, and add the noodles.

Variation:

Replacing the butternut squash with zucchini noodles or shirataki noodles (usually found in the produce section of the grocery store) will lower the carbohydrate count in this recipe.

Per Serving: Calories: 175; Total fat: 7g; Saturated fat: 1g; Sodium: 159mg; Total carbohydrates: 22g; Sugar: 5g; Fiber: 4g; Net carbohydrates: 18g; Protein: 4g

Tofu Veggie Stir-Fry

30 MINUTES OR LESS, GLUTEN-FREE, NUT-FREE, ONE-POT, VEGAN

Serves 3
Prep time: 10 minutes

Cook time: 20 minutes

Who needs takeout? This heart-healthy, high-fiber stir-fry is fragrant with ginger and garlic. Cauliflower rice in place of the usual white rice make this recipe especially healthy. You can easily make your own cauliflower rice using the instructions on page 213, or you can find it premade in many supermarkets.

- 2 tablespoons extra-virgin olive oil
- 4 scallions, sliced
- 12 ounces firm tofu, cut into ½-inch pieces
- 4 cups broccoli, broken into florets
- 4 garlic cloves, minced
- 1 teaspoon peeled and grated fresh ginger
- ¼ cup vegetable broth
- 2 tablespoons soy sauce (use gluten-free soy sauce if necessary)
- 1 cup Cauliflower Rice (page 213)

1. In a large skillet over medium-high heat, heat the olive oil until it shimmers. Add the scallions, tofu, and broccoli and cook, stirring, until the vegetables begin to soften, about 6 minutes. Add the garlic and ginger and cook, stirring constantly, for 30 seconds.
2. Add the vegetable broth, soy sauce, and cauliflower rice. Cook, stirring, 1 to 2 minutes more to heat the rice through.

Storage Tip:

Refrigerate in a sealed container for up to 5 days or freeze for up to 6 months.

Per Serving: Calories: 320; Total fat: 20g; Saturated fat: 3g; Sodium: 412mg; Total carbohydrates: 19g; Sugar: 3g; Fiber: 7g; Net carbohydrates: 12g; Protein: 24g

Tabbouleh Pita

30 MINUTES OR LESS, NUT-FREE, SOY-FREE, VEGAN

Serves 4   **Prep time:** 20 minutes

Tabbouleh is a popular Middle Eastern salad made with tomatoes, parsley, and cooked bulgur wheat or couscous as the base. Stuffing pitas with this complex and colorful mixture is a marvelous way to enjoy the taste and health benefits of all these foods on the go. Make sure you get pitas that are designed for stuffing with hearty fillings, because some products do not open easily and are better suited for dipping into hummus.

4 whole wheat pitas

1 cup cooked bulgur wheat

1 English cucumber, finely chopped

2 cups halved cherry tomatoes

1 yellow bell pepper, seeded and finely chopped

2 scallions, white and green parts, finely chopped

½ cup finely chopped fresh parsley

2 tablespoons extra-virgin olive oil

Juice of 1 lemon

Kosher salt

Freshly ground black pepper

1. Cut the pitas in half and split them open. Set them aside.
2. In a large bowl, stir together the bulgur, cucumber, tomatoes, bell pepper, scallions, parsley, olive oil, and lemon juice.
3. Season the bulgur mixture with salt and pepper.
4. Spoon the bulgur mixture evenly into the pita halves and serve.

Per Serving: Calories: 242; Total fat: 8g; Saturated fat: 2g; Sodium: 164mg; Total carbohydrates: 39g; Sugar: 4g; Fiber: 6g; Net carbohydrates: 33g; Protein: 7g

Gingered Red Lentils with Millet

30 MINUTES OR LESS, GLUTEN-FREE, SOY-FREE, VEGAN

Serves 4
Prep time: 10 minutes

Cook time: 20 minutes

This recipe is inspired by Indian dal. Cooks in India long ago mastered the art of balanced eating and embraced the understanding that you don't have to sacrifice great bold flavors to enjoy vegetarian food. You will find the blend of ginger, mint, onions, and tomato in this dish is, in a word, perfect.

2 cups water

½ cup millet, rinsed

½ cup red
  lentils, rinsed

1 tablespoon
  extra-virgin olive oil

Pinch kosher salt

1 onion, diced

3-inch piece ginger,
  grated (or minced)

4 cups cherry toma-
  toes, quartered

3 tablespoons unsalted
  peanuts, chopped

2 limes, quartered

1 bunch mint leaves

1. In a medium saucepan over medium heat, stir together the water, millet, lentils, and salt. Bring to a boil, reduce the heat to low, cover, and simmer until tender, about 15 minutes. Remove the saucepan from the heat and let the grains sit for a few minutes.

2. Meanwhile, in a small saucepan, heat the olive oil over a medium heat. Sauté the onion until translucent, about 3 minutes. Add the ginger, tomatoes, and peanuts. Cook for about 5 minutes, adjust the seasonings as desired, and allow to sit until the millet and lentils are finished.

3. Divide the millet and lentils among four bowls and top them with the gingered onion mixture. Garnish with lime wedges and mint leaves.

Storage Tip:

Store any leftovers in an airtight container in the refrigerator for up to 3 days.

Per Serving: Calories: 288; Total fat: 9g; Saturated fat: 1g; Sodium: 51mg; Total carbohydrates: 44g; Sugar: 6g; Fiber: 8g; Net carbohydrates: 36g; Protein: 12g

Peanut Tofu over Buckwheat Noodles

30 MINUTES OR LESS, VEGAN

Serves 2
Prep time: 5 to 10 minutes

Cook time: 10 minutes

This delightful recipe is loaded with veggies, enough for your entire day, as well as deliciously thick buckwheat noodles. Yes, you can eat noodles if you're a diabetic or are trying to limit your carbohydrates; this recipe simply ensures that you're not getting too much of a good thing.

1½ ounces buckwheat noodles

¼ cup Peanut Sauce (page 216) or store-bought

4 cups shredded cabbage

8 ounces firm tofu, cubed

1 cup diced cucumber

½ cup chopped cilantro

1. Cook the buckwheat noodles according to the package instructions and allow to cool. This can be done 1 to 2 days in advance, and you can store the cooked noodles in the refrigerator in an airtight container.
2. In a large bowl, thin the peanut sauce with water if it's too thick. It should resemble the consistency of a thin dressing. Toss the sauce with the noodles, cabbage, tofu, cucumber, and cilantro. Adjust the seasonings as desired. Serve.

Storage Tip:

Store any leftovers in an airtight container in the refrigerator for up to 3 days.

Variation:

If you like extra sauce, double up on the peanut sauce. It will increase your protein and fat to keep you fuller longer. If you're not a fan of cilantro, you can use equal amounts of parsley, any lettuce, red cabbage, or shredded carrot instead.

Per Serving: Calories: 371; Total fat: 17g; Saturated fat: 3g; Sodium: 540mg; Total carbohydrates: 35g; Sugar: 8g; Fiber: 9g; Net carbohydrates: 26g; Protein: 26g

Eggplant and Lentils with Curried Yogurt

GLUTEN-FREE, SOY-FREE, VEGETARIAN

Serves 4

Prep time: 10 minutes

Cook time: 45 minutes

This dish is a crowd-pleasing recipe that'll be devoured at your next family dinner or neighborhood potluck. If you have the time before you begin cooking, soaking the lentils for 1 hour before preparing this dish helps shorten the cooking time.

2 large eggplants

4 tablespoons extra-virgin olive oil, divided

Kosher salt

2 cups water

¾ cup brown lentils, rinsed and soaked (optional to soak)

1 teaspoon ground cumin, divided

¾ cup plain nonfat Greek yogurt

2 teaspoons curry powder

Juice and grated zest of 1 lime

1 onion, thinly sliced

¼ cup sliced almonds

½ teaspoon ground coriander

¼ cup pomegranate arils

1. Preheat the oven to 450°F. Line a baking sheet with parchment paper.
2. Use a peeler to peel strips of the skin off the eggplant lengthwise. Alternate strips, leaving some of the purplish-black skin on the eggplant. It should be reminiscent of a zebra with the white flesh and dark skin. Cut the peeled eggplant width-wise into ½-inch-thick slices. Place them in a medium bowl.
3. Toss the eggplant with 2 tablespoons of olive oil and a pinch of salt. Spread the slices in a single layer on the prepared baking sheet. Roast the eggplant for 20 minutes, until slightly crispy and soft.
4. Meanwhile, in a medium stockpot over medium-high heat, combine the water, lentils, ½ teaspoon of cumin, and a pinch of salt. Bring to a boil, then reduce the heat to low, cover, and simmer for 20 minutes or until the lentils are tender. Set aside.
5. In a small bowl, combine the Greek yogurt with the curry powder, 1 tablespoon of lime juice, and a pinch of lime zest. Taste and adjust the seasonings as desired. Use the additional lime juice if you feel it should have more citrus or a looser consistency. Set aside.
6. In a medium skillet over medium-high heat, heat the remaining 2 tablespoons of olive oil. Sauté the onion until translucent, about 3 minutes. Add the remaining ½ teaspoon of cumin, the sliced almonds, and coriander to the skillet, stirring to combine.

7. Arrange the slices of eggplant on four plates, followed by the lentils, spiced yogurt, and sautéed onions, and garnish with pomegranate arils.

Variation:

You can use dried cherries or dried cranberries in place of the pomegranate arils, if preferred.

Per Serving: Calories: 399; Total fat: 17g; Saturated fat: 2g; Sodium: 64mg; Total carbohydrates: 45g; Sugar: 15g; Fiber: 14g; Net carbohydrates: 31g; Protein: 19g

Simple Bibimbap

30 MINUTES OR LESS, DAIRY-FREE, NUT-FREE, VEGETARIAN

Serves 2

Prep time: 15 minutes

Cook time: 15 minutes

Korean-inspired bibimbap ("bibim" means to mix various ingredients and "bap" means rice) is the ultimate casual meal. Feel free to experiment with the extra veggies and sauces you have in the refrigerator as well. The cauliflower rice helps you cut back on the concentrated carbs of traditional rice, and kimchi is a delicious good-for-your-gut probiotic food that helps with digestion and immunity. You can find it at many grocery stores in the international aisle.

4 teaspoons avocado oil, divided

2½ cups Cauliflower Rice (page 213)

2 cups fresh baby spinach

1 tablespoon reduced-sodium soy sauce or tamari, divided

8 ounces mushrooms, thinly sliced

2 large eggs

1 cup bean sprouts, rinsed

1 cup kimchi

½ cup shredded carrots

1. In a medium skillet over a medium heat, heat 1 teaspoon of avocado oil and sauté the cauliflower rice, spinach, and 2 teaspoons of soy sauce until the greens are wilted, about 5 minutes. Put the vegetables in a small bowl and set aside.

2. Return the skillet to medium heat, add 2 teaspoons of avocado oil, and, when it's hot, add the mushrooms in a single layer and cook for 3 to 5 minutes, then stir and cook another 3 minutes or until mostly golden-brown in color. Put the mushrooms in a small bowl and toss them with the remaining 1 teaspoon of soy sauce.

3. Wipe out the skillet and heat the remaining 1 teaspoon of avocado oil over low heat. Crack in the eggs and cook until the whites are set and the yolks begin to thicken but not harden, 4 to 5 minutes.

4. Assemble two bowls with cauliflower rice and spinach at the bottom. Then arrange each ingredient separately around the rim of the bowl: bean sprouts, mushrooms, kimchi, and shredded carrots, with the egg placed in the center, and serve.

Variation:

Add some sliced radishes for more vegetables or serve with whole grains.

Per Serving: Calories: 277; Total fat: 15g; Saturated fat: 3g; Sodium: 548mg; Total carbohydrates: 20g; Sugar: 7g; Fiber: 8g; Net carbohydrates: 12g; Protein: 18g

Jackfruit Tacos

30 MINUTES OR LESS, GLUTEN-FREE, NUT-FREE, VEGAN

Serves 4
Prep time: 5 minutes

Cook time: 25 minutes

You may have heard of jackfruit as the go-to meat substitute. Not only does it have a succulent texture like that of pulled pork, but it also takes on the flavor and spice of ingredients it's cooked with. Surprisingly, jackfruit is best canned as opposed to raw. You can find it in Asian markets or the international aisle of your grocery store.

1 (20-ounce) can jack-fruit in water, rinsed and drained

2 tablespoons extra-virgin olive oil

1 yellow onion, diced

1 cup water

4 garlic cloves, minced

2 teaspoons paprika

1 tablespoon chili powder

1 tablespoon ground cumin

1 chipotle pepper in adobo sauce, minced, plus 2 tablespoons sauce

Juice of 2 limes

Corn tortillas

Optional toppings

Shredded cabbage or lettuce

Salsa

Cooked beans

Avocado

1. Place the jackfruit in a medium bowl. Sort through it and cut the tougher core portion of the jackfruit into smaller pieces. Use your hands to break up some of the larger, tender pieces. Pat dry and set aside.

2. In a large skillet over medium heat, heat the olive oil and sauté the onion until translucent, 3 to 5 minutes. Add the jackfruit, water, garlic, paprika, chili powder, cumin, chipotle pepper and adobo sauce, and lime juice. Mix well, reduce the heat to medium-low, cover, and cook, stirring occasionally, for 15 minutes.

3. Serve with corn tortillas, lettuce or cabbage, and any other taco additions you see fit.

Storage Tip:

Refrigerate any leftovers in an airtight container for up to 4 days.

Per Serving: Calories: 231; Total fat: 8g; Saturated fat: 1g; Sodium: 65mg; Total carbohydrates: 41g; Sugar: 29g; Fiber: 4g; Net carbohydrates: 37g; Protein: 4g

Acorn Squash Stuffed with Tofu and Apple

GLUTEN-FREE, VEGAN

Serves 4

Prep time: 15 minutes

Cook time: 40 minutes

This meatless stuffed acorn squash is so flavorful and filling! The tofu absorbs the apple and raisin flavors in the oven. Cooking the squash first lets it get tender before the quicker-cooking ingredients are added.

2 large acorn squash, halved and seeded

1 (14-ounce) package firm tofu, drained

1 apple (unpeeled), cored and cut into ½-inch cubes

⅓ cup raisins

2 tablespoons chopped walnuts

Shelled pumpkin seeds, for garnish (optional)

1. Preheat the oven to 375°F.
2. Place the 4 acorn squash halves on a half sheet pan, cut-side down. Bake for 25 minutes.
3. While the squash is baking, pat the tofu dry with paper towels and cut into 1-inch cubes. Combine the tofu, apple, raisins, and walnuts in a bowl.
4. Turn the squash halves over and fill each with the tofu mixture. Bake for 15 minutes.
5. Garnish with pumpkin seeds, if desired.

Variation:

You can make this with chunks of cooked turkey instead of tofu.

Per Serving: Calories: 313; Total fat: 11g; Saturated fat: 2g; Sodium: 24mg; Total carbohydrates: 43g; Fiber: 7g; Sugar: 12g; Net carbohydrates: 36g; Protein: 12g

Cauliflower Steaks with Tomato, Caper, and Golden Raisin Sauce

30 MINUTES OR LESS, GLUTEN-FREE, NUT-FREE, SOY-FREE, VEGAN

Serves 4
Prep time: 5 minutes

Cook time: 25 minutes

If you've never tried a cauliflower steak, now is the time. This version includes a stellar sauce made with tomatoes, capers, and golden raisins. This Italian-influenced plate will linger in your memory long after the last bite.

1 large head cauliflower	2 tablespoons extra-virgin olive oil Pinch kosher salt	Pinch freshly ground black pepper	1 batch Tomato, Caper, and Golden Raisin Sauce (page 221)

1. Preheat the oven to 400°F. Line a baking sheet with parchment paper.
2. Stand up the cauliflower so that the stem end is flat on the cutting board while you hold the crown of the head with your hand. Then, carefully, slice ½-inch-thick "steaks" starting from the crown (top of the head) and moving toward the stem (base). Work from one end to the other. Depending on the size of the cauliflower, you should get 4 to 6 sliced steaks and some florets.
3. Place the cauliflower steaks and florets on the prepared baking sheet in a single layer. Brush them with olive oil and season with salt and pepper.
4. Roast the cauliflower for 15 minutes until golden brown, then flip the steaks over and cook for another 10 minutes.
5. To serve, lay the cauliflower steaks on plates and top with the tomato sauce.

Storage Tip:

Store any leftovers in an airtight container in the refrigerator for up to 4 days.

Prep Tip:

If you really want to cut down on the cooking time, you can always use a canned tomato sauce instead of making the tomato-caper sauce. Simply heat the sauce in a saucepan on the stove until warm.

Per Serving: Calories: 210; Total fat: 9g; Saturated fat: 3g; Sodium: 243mg; Total carbohydrates: 22g; Sugar: 10g; Fiber: 6g; Net carbohydrates: 16g; Protein: 7g

Veggie Unfried Rice

DAIRY-FREE, GLUTEN-FREE, SOY-FREE, VEGETARIAN

Serves 4
Prep time: 15 minutes

Cook time: 25 minutes

There is almost nothing better than a well-seasoned vegetable rice, a balanced dish with protein, heart-healthy fats, and complex carbohydrates all in one. The collard greens are the standout here, providing color contrast and a satisfyingly pungent taste. Feel free to try duck or quail eggs instead of the traditional chicken egg.

1 tablespoon extra-virgin olive oil

1 bunch collard greens, stemmed and cut into chiffonade

½ cup Vegetable Broth (page 225) or store-bought low-sodium vegetable broth

1 carrot, cut into 2-inch matchsticks

1 red onion, thinly sliced

1 garlic clove, minced

2 tablespoons reduced-sodium soy sauce

2 cups riced cauliflower or butternut squash

1 large egg

1 teaspoon red pepper flakes

1 teaspoon paprika

1. In a large Dutch oven, heat the olive oil over medium heat.
2. Add the collard greens and cook for 3 to 5 minutes, or until the greens are wilted.
3. Add the broth, carrot, onion, garlic, and soy sauce, then cover and cook for 5 to 7 minutes, or until the carrot softens and the onion and garlic are translucent.
4. Uncover, add the riced vegetable, and cook for 2 to 3 minutes, gently mixing all the ingredients together until well combined but not mushy.
5. Crack the egg over the pot and gently scramble the egg. Cook for 2 to 5 minutes, or until the egg is no longer runny.
6. Remove from the heat and season with the red pepper flakes and paprika.

Per Serving (2 cups): Calories: 100; Total fat: 5g; Saturated fat: 1g; Sodium: 309mg; Total carbohydrates: 10g; Sugar: 3g; Fiber: 4g; Net carbohydrates: 6g; Protein: 6g

Baked Egg Skillet with Avocado

30 MINUTES OR LESS, DAIRY-FREE, GLUTEN-FREE, NUT-FREE, ONE-POT, SOY-FREE, VEGETARIAN

Serves 4
Prep time: 5 minutes

Cook time: 25 minutes

With its lovely Southwestern flavor profile, these eggs are great for a family dinner. You can add additional non-starchy veggies, such as spinach, kale, or red bell peppers, for additional vitamins and minerals. You can also replace the avocado with homemade guacamole.

2 tablespoons extra-virgin olive oil

1 red onion, chopped

1 green bell pepper, seeded and chopped

1 sweet potato, cut into ½-inch pieces

1 teaspoon chili powder

½ teaspoon kosher salt

4 medium eggs

1 avocado, cut into cubes

1. Preheat the oven to 350°F.
2. In a large, ovenproof skillet over medium-high heat, heat the olive oil until it shimmers. Add the onion, bell pepper, sweet potato, chili powder, and salt, and cook, stirring occasionally, until the vegetables start to brown, about 10 minutes.
3. Remove from the heat. Arrange the vegetables in the pan to form 4 wells. Crack an egg into each well and bake until the eggs set, about 10 minutes.
4. Top with avocado before serving.

Storage Tip:

This won't keep well. Make it fresh and enjoy it right away.

Variation:

For fewer carbs, you can replace the sweet potato with 1 cup of raw chopped carrots, which has only about 5 grams of carbs per serving. For a few extra grams of carbs, you can top each serving with 2 tablespoons of prepared salsa. Check the serving size and carbohydrate counts on the salsa and look for products with less than 5 grams of sugar. You can also add chopped tomatoes to serve.

Per Serving: Calories: 250; Total fat: 18g; Saturated fat: 3g; Sodium: 251mg; Total carbohydrates: 16g; Sugar: 4g; Fiber: 5g; Net carbohydrates: 11g; Protein: 8g

Veggie Chili

30 MINUTES OR LESS, NUT-FREE, ONE-POT, VEGAN

Serves 4   Cook time: 15 minutes
Prep time: 10 minutes

This combination of beans and vegetarian proteins is hearty and nutritious. In addition to the protein, it's packed with low-glycemic carbohydrates and contains calcium and iron. You can find veggie crumbles in the freezer section of many grocery stores. Double-check the label for the exact grams of carbs per serving and take this into account if you vary this recipe.

2 tablespoons extra-virgin olive oil

1 onion, finely chopped

1 green bell pepper, seeded and chopped

2 (14-ounce) cans crushed tomatoes

1 (14-ounce) can kidney beans, drained and rinsed

2 cups veggie crumbles (such as MorningStar Farms Grillers Crumbles)

1 tablespoon chili powder

1 teaspoon garlic powder

½ teaspoon kosher salt

1. In a large skillet over medium-high heat, heat the olive oil until it shimmers. Add the onion and bell pepper and cook, stirring occasionally, for 5 minutes.
2. Add the tomatoes, beans, veggie crumbles, chili powder, garlic powder, and salt. Bring to a simmer, stirring. Reduce heat and cook for 5 minutes more, stirring occasionally.

Storage Tip:

Refrigerate in a sealed container for up to 3 days or freeze for up to 6 months.

Variation:

Reduce carbs by about 11 grams per serving by reducing kidney beans to ½ can. Add 4 cups of vegetable broth to make a chili soup.

Per Serving: Calories: 283; Total fat: 10g; Saturated fat: 1g; Sodium: 780mg; Total carbohydrates: 39g; Sugar: 14g; Fiber: 13g; Net carbohydrates: 26g; Protein: 17g

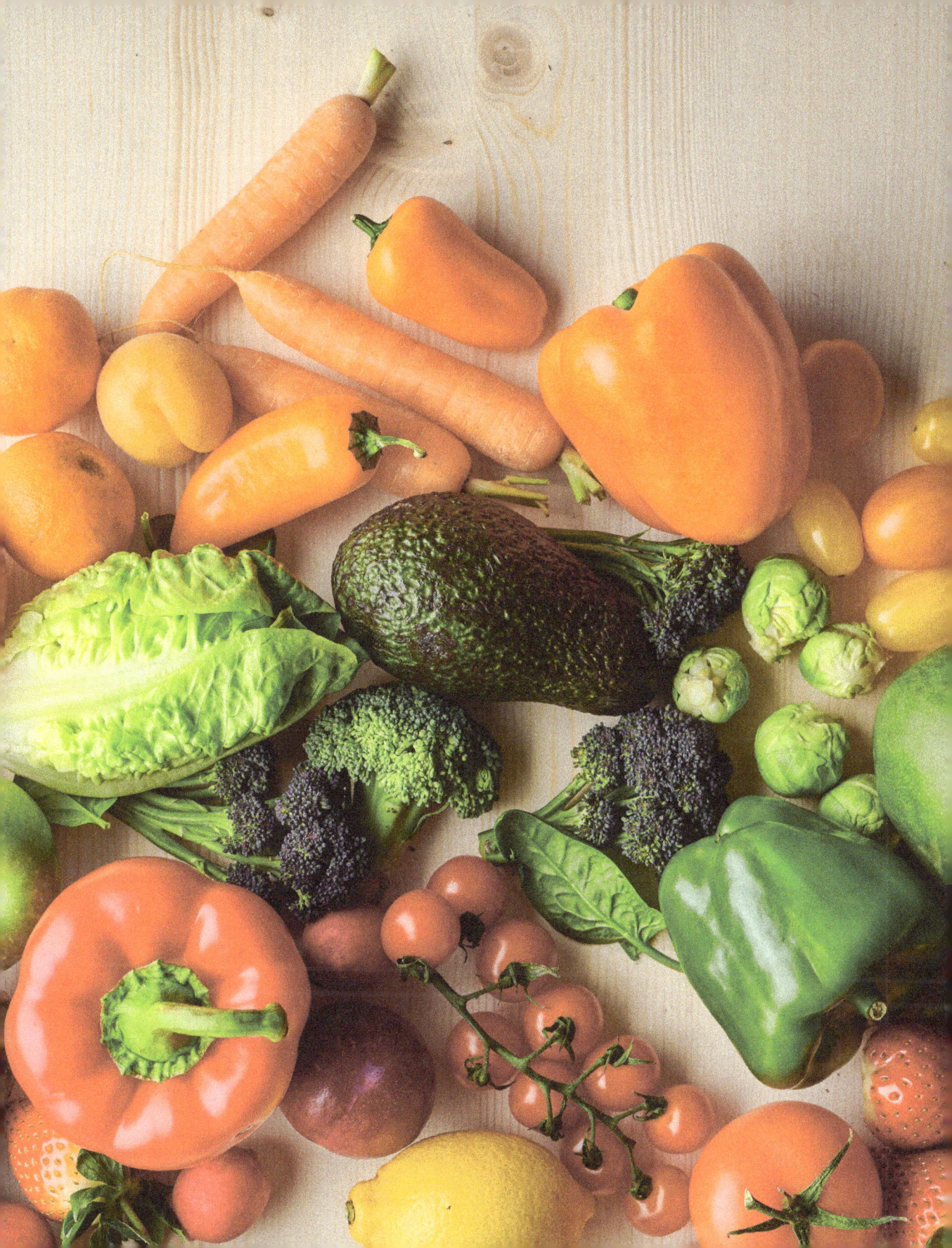

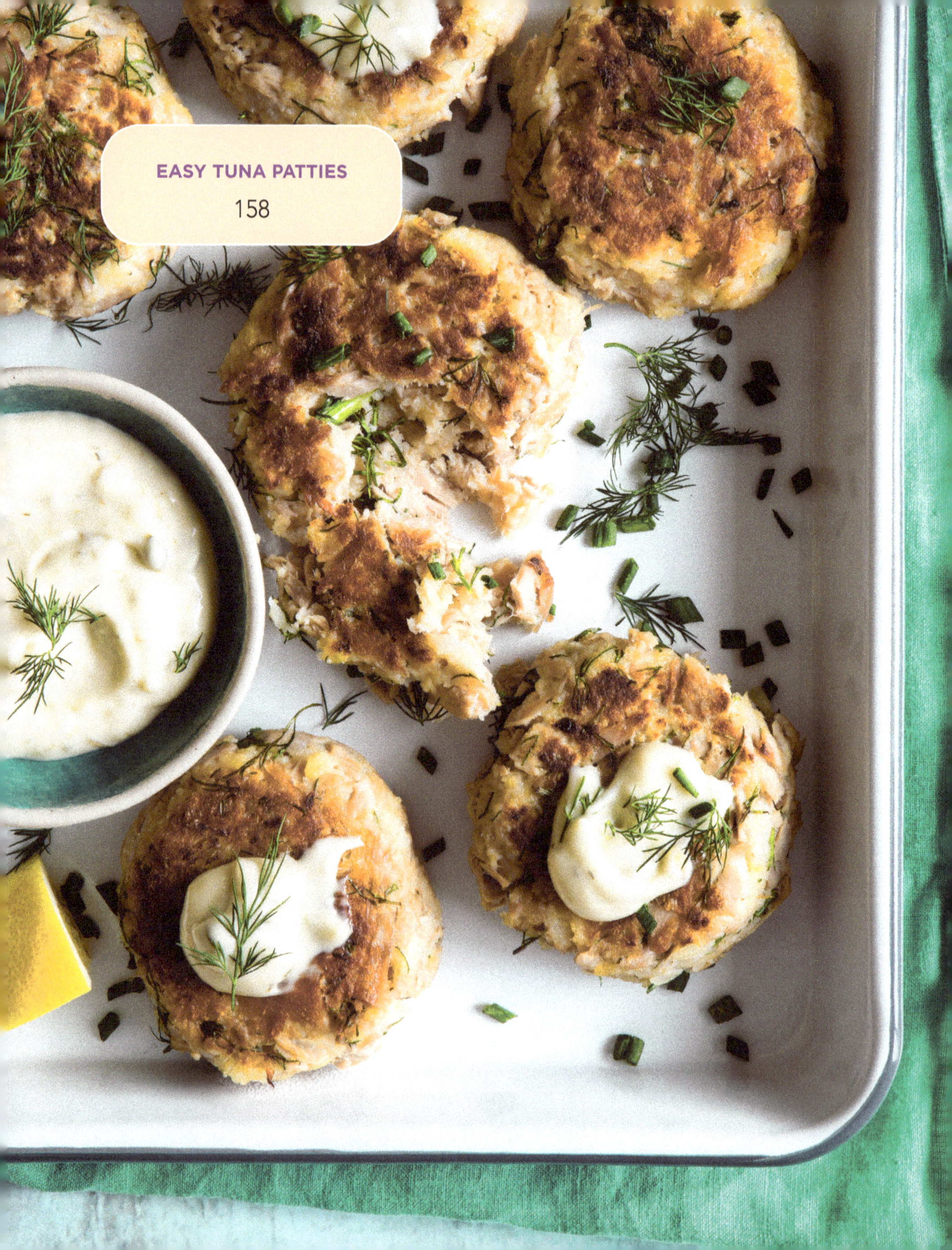

EASY TUNA PATTIES

158

6

POULTRY AND FISH

Stewed Herbed Whole Chicken with California Vegetables

DAIRY-FREE, GLUTEN-FREE, NUT-FREE, ONE-POT, SOY-FREE

Serves 4
Prep time: 10 minutes

Cook time: 1 hour 15 minutes

Cooking a whole chicken in the Dutch oven is super easy and leaves you with delicious leftovers for later in the week. You can use the carcass to make your own chicken stock when you have the time. Until then, put the bones in a freezer bag and keep for up to four months. Toss the giblets in there, too (except the liver); they'll add flavor to your stock.

1 whole chicken (about 4 pounds), giblets removed

1 teaspoon minced garlic

1 teaspoon freshly ground black pepper

1 teaspoon poultry seasoning

1 teaspoon dried parsley

1 (24-ounce) package frozen California vegetable blend

1. In a Dutch oven, place the chicken breast-side up. Rub the chicken breast and legs with the garlic, pepper, poultry seasoning, and parsley.
2. Add water until it's 1 inch from the top of the pot. Bring the water to a slow boil over medium-low heat, for about 10 minutes. Cover, reduce the heat, and simmer for 45 to 60 minutes. To ensure the chicken is completely cooked, insert a meat thermometer in the thickest part of the breast. The meat is cooked when the thermometer reads 165°F.
3. Transfer the chicken to a cutting board and let it rest for 5 minutes before cutting to avoid the loss of juices. Add the frozen vegetables to the broth in the pot and cook until heated through, about 5 minutes. Remove the vegetables with a slotted spoon to serve (and reserve the broth for another use). Serve chicken skinless with a generous side of vegetables.

Storage Tip:

Refrigerate the leftover cooked chicken pieces in an airtight container for up to 2 days or freeze for up to 9 months. A whole cooked chicken can be frozen for up to 1 year.

Per Serving (6 ounces skinless chicken and ¼ veggies): Calories: 314; Total fat: 6g; Saturated fat: 1g; Sodium: 208mg; Total carbohydrates: 23g; Sugar: 1g; Fiber: 7g; Net carbohydrates: 16g; Protein: 40g

Herb-Roasted Chicken Breast

30 MINUTES OR LESS, DAIRY-FREE, GLUTEN-FREE, NUT-FREE, SOY-FREE

Serves 4
Prep time: 5 minutes

Cook time: 25 minutes

You know how bland, dry, overcooked chicken is no one's favorite? This recipe takes care of that. This easy meal uses key herbs and spices to create extremely juicy, flavorful chicken your family will love. Choose chicken breasts of equal size so they cook more evenly and serve with a colorful side of steamed veggies such as asparagus, broccoli, or carrots.

1 tablespoon
  extra-virgin olive oil

1 teaspoon chopped
  fresh thyme

½ teaspoon
  dried oregano

½ teaspoon
  garlic powder

½ teaspoon
  onion powder

½ teaspoon kosher salt

4 (4-ounce) bone-
  less, skinless
  chicken breasts

1. Preheat the oven to 400°F.
2. In a small bowl, stir together the olive oil, thyme, oregano, garlic powder, onion powder, and salt.
3. Place the chicken breasts on a baking sheet or in a baking dish and rub both sides with the herb mixture. Leave a couple of inches between each breast. Bake for 20 to 25 minutes, until the juices run clear and the internal temperature measures 165°F on an instant-read thermometer.
4. Let the chicken rest for 5 minutes before slicing and serving.

Prep Tip:

When cooking chicken breasts, which tend to dry out easily, having uniformly sized pieces helps with even cooking. If any of your chicken breasts are thicker than about ¾ inch, place them on a cutting board, cover with plastic wrap, and pound with a kitchen mallet until about ¾-inch thick.

Per Serving: Calories: 140; Total fat: 4g; Saturated fat: 1g; Sodium: 243mg; Total carbohydrates: 1g; Sugar: 0g; Fiber: 0g; Net carbohydrates: 1g; Protein: 24g

Baked Chicken Tenders

30 MINUTES OR LESS, DAIRY-FREE, NUT-FREE, SOY-FREE

Serves 4

Prep time: 10 minutes

Cook time: 15 minutes

Cutting chicken into ½-inch-thick pieces and pounding it slightly so that the pieces are the same thickness helps it cook evenly. By choosing breast meat rather than the thigh, you get a much leaner protein source.

- 1 cup whole wheat bread crumbs
- 1 tablespoon dried thyme
- 1 teaspoon garlic powder
- 1 teaspoon paprika
- ½ teaspoon kosher salt
- 3 large eggs, beaten
- 1 tablespoon Dijon mustard
- 1 pound chicken, cut into ½-inch-thick pieces and pounded to even thickness

1. Preheat the oven to 375°F. Line a rimmed baking sheet with parchment paper.
2. In a medium bowl, whisk together the bread crumbs, thyme, garlic powder, paprika, and salt.
3. In another bowl, whisk together the eggs and mustard.
4. Dip each piece of chicken in the egg mixture, then in the bread crumb mixture. Place on the prepared baking sheet.
5. Bake until the chicken reaches an internal temperature of 165°F and the bread crumbs are golden, about 15 minutes.

Storage Tip:

Refrigerate in a sealed container for up to 3 days or freeze for up to 6 months. Reheat in a 375°F oven for about 15 minutes.

Variation:

Serve these tenders on a bed of greens as a salad or enjoy each serving with 1 cup of cooked sweet potato, which adds an estimated 30 grams of carbohydrates.

Per Serving: Calories: 276; Total fat: 6g; Saturated fat: 2g; Sodium: 487mg; Total carbohydrates: 17g; Sugar: 2g; Fiber: 3g; Net carbohydrates: 14g; Protein: 34g

Chicken with Lemon Caper Pan Sauce

30 MINUTES OR LESS, GLUTEN-FREE, NUT-FREE, SOY-FREE

Serves 4
Prep time: 10 minutes

Cook time: 15 minutes

Pound the chicken breast slightly between two pieces of plastic wrap to an even thickness so the chicken cooks evenly. The lemon caper sauce adds tasty elements of salt and acid to the sweet flavor of the chicken.

2 tablespoons extra-virgin olive oil

4 (5-ounce) boneless, skinless chicken breasts, halved lengthwise and pounded slightly to even thickness

½ teaspoon kosher salt
⅛ teaspoon freshly ground black pepper
¼ cup freshly squeezed lemon juice

¼ cup dry white wine
2 tablespoons capers, rinsed
1 tablespoon salted butter, very cold, cut into pieces

1. In a large skillet over medium-high heat, heat the olive oil until it shimmers.
2. Season the chicken with the salt and pepper. Add it to the hot oil and cook until opaque with an internal temperature of 165°F, about 5 minutes per side. Transfer the chicken to a plate and tent loosely with foil to keep warm. Keep the pan on the heat.
3. Add the lemon juice and wine to the pan, using the side of a spoon to scrape any browned bits from the bottom of the pan. Add the capers. Simmer until the liquid is reduced by half, about 3 minutes. Reduce the heat to low.
4. Whisk in the butter, one piece at a time, until incorporated.
5. Return the chicken to the pan, turning once to coat with the sauce. Serve with additional sauce spooned over the top.

Storage Tip:

Refrigerate for up to 3 days, storing the sauce separately from the chicken.

Per Serving: Calories: 244; Total fat: 12g; Saturated fat: 3g; Sodium: 274mg; Total carbohydrates: 2g; Sugar: 0g; Fiber: <1g; Net carbohydrates: 2g; Protein: 26g

Chicken Ratatouille

DAIRY-FREE, GLUTEN-FREE, NUT-FREE, ONE-POT, SOY-FREE

Serves 4
Prep time: 15 minutes

Cook time: 25 minutes

Ratatouille is a classic French dish. It combines a mix of stewed vegetables, usually eggplant, zucchini, peppers, and tomatoes, for a variety of colors and textures. In this version, shredded chicken is used to balance out the bowl with a protein. If you want a gluten-free version, be sure to check the label of the stewed tomatoes or use diced tomatoes instead.

2 tablespoons extra-virgin olive oil

1 large onion, chopped

2 cups low-sodium vegetable broth

2 large eggplants, cut into 1-inch chunks

2 carrots, sliced

1 large zucchini, sliced

1 large red bell pepper, seeded and coarsely chopped

1 (28-ounce) can reduced-sodium stewed tomatoes

1 teaspoon dried thyme, plus more for garnish (optional)

1 (12½-ounce) can chunk chicken or 2½ cups chopped cooked chicken

1. Preheat the oven to 400°F.
2. In a Dutch oven over medium heat, heat the olive oil until it shimmers. Add the onion and sauté until tender, about 3 minutes.
3. Add the broth, eggplants, carrots, zucchini, bell pepper, tomatoes with their juices, and thyme and mix well. Stir in the chicken.
4. Cover and bake for 20 minutes, until all the vegetables are tender.
5. Sprinkle dried thyme on top as a garnish, if desired.

Per Serving: Calories: 348; Total fat: 11g; Saturated fat: 1g; Sodium: 309mg; Total carbohydrates: 39g; Sugar: 21g; Fiber: 16g; Net carbohydrates: 21g; Protein: 30g

Braised Chicken Stew

DAIRY-FREE, NUT-FREE, ONE-POT, SOY-FREE

Serves 4
Prep time: 30 minutes

Cook time: 1 hour

This comfort food will warm you up any time of the year, and it's budget-friendly. Chicken legs are inexpensive and can be bought in bulk. You can store them in the freezer in the original package for a short time, but it's best to repackage them in plastic wrap and airtight freezer bags.

- 1 tablespoon avocado oil or extra-virgin olive oil
- 3 pounds bone-in, skin-on chicken thighs and drumsticks, trimmed of excess skin and fat
- ½ teaspoon poultry seasoning
- 1 medium onion, chopped
- 2 carrots, thinly sliced
- 1 celery stalk, thinly sliced on the diagonal
- 2 tablespoons all-purpose flour
- 1 (28-ounce) can reduced-sodium diced tomatoes
- 1 (4-ounce) can sliced mushrooms, drained
- 2 large sweet potatoes, peeled and cut into 1-inch chunks
- ½ teaspoon dried thyme
- 1 bay leaf
- 4 cups low-sodium chicken broth

1. In a large Dutch oven over medium heat, heat the avocado oil until it shimmers. Add the chicken pieces, skin-side down, and brown them for 3 minutes. Turn the chicken pieces over.
2. Add the poultry seasoning, onion, carrots, and celery and cook for about 5 minutes. Stir in the flour and mix well.
3. Add the tomatoes with their juices, mushrooms, sweet potatoes, thyme, and bay leaf and mix well. Stir in the broth.
4. Bring the stew to a boil, then cover and simmer, stirring occasionally, for about 45 minutes, until the vegetables and chicken are thoroughly cooked.

Per Serving: Calories: 474; Total fat: 20g; Saturated fat: 1g; Sodium: 156mg; Total carbohydrates: 30g; Sugar: 12g; Fiber: 5g; Net carbohydrates: 25g; Protein: 49g

Panko Chicken Potpie

NUT-FREE, ONE-POT, SOY-FREE

Serves 4

Prep time: 15 minutes

Cook time: 30 minutes

Making and eating a homemade version of potpie doesn't have to be difficult. Potpie generally has a protein stuffing of beef, chicken, turkey, or seafood and both a top and a bottom crust. This easy meal includes only a top crust and a variety of vegetables, plus some chicken, to give you a well-balanced meal that doesn't take all day in the kitchen.

Nonstick cooking spray

1 (12½-ounce) can chunk chicken or 2½ cups chopped cooked chicken

1 (12-ounce) package frozen mixed vegetables (no need to thaw)

1 (15-ounce) can lima beans, rinsed and drained

1 (12-ounce) jar or can reduced-sodium chicken gravy

1 teaspoon freshly ground black pepper

1 teaspoon dried tarragon

½ cup panko bread crumbs

½ cup grated Parmesan cheese

1. Preheat the oven to 375°F. Spray a casserole dish with nonstick cooking spray.
2. Combine the chicken, mixed vegetables, lima beans, gravy, pepper, and tarragon in the casserole dish and mix well.
3. Sprinkle the panko bread crumbs and Parmesan cheese over the top.
4. Cover and bake for 30 minutes, or until the mixture begins to bubble.

Variation:

If you would like to make this gluten-free, substitute toasted quinoa or riced cauliflower for the panko bread crumbs. If you don't have chicken on hand but have leftover beef strips, pulled pork, or salmon, you can change up the filling and create your own special potpie.

Per Serving: Calories: 433; Total fat: 11g; Saturated fat: 3g; Sodium: 471mg; Total carbohydrates: 40g; Sugar: 3g; Fiber: 10g; Net carbohydrates: 30g; Protein: 36g

Barbecue Chicken

DAIRY-FREE, GLUTEN-FREE, NUT-FREE, SOY-FREE

Serves 4
Prep time: 10 minutes

Cook time: 25 minutes

Barbecue chicken is a classic summer meal for a reason. But when it's a bit too cold to fire up the grill, oven-barbecued chicken is the perfect solution. It pairs well with greens and skillet corn bread, and you'll almost feel the sun on your face as you dig in.

4 boneless, skinless chicken thighs	1 tablespoon smoked paprika	1 cup Barbecue Sauce (page 215)	Freshly ground black pepper

1. Preheat the oven to 375°F.
2. In a small mixing bowl, combine the chicken, paprika, and barbecue sauce, coating the chicken thoroughly. Set aside for 15 minutes.
3. Place the chicken in a cast-iron skillet in a single layer.
4. Transfer the skillet to the oven and cook for 25 minutes, or until the juices from the chicken run clear.
5. Season with black pepper and serve.

Variation:

If you haven't made your own barbecue sauce, substitute a store-bought version. Ideally, look for one with limited additives and preservatives, and find those with limited added sugars, salts, and fats.

Per Serving (1 thigh): Calories: 229; Total fat: 5g; Saturated fat: 1g; Sodium: 199mg; Total carbohydrates: 10g; Sugar: 4g; Fiber: 2g; Net carbohydrates: 8g; Protein: 23g

Skillet-Blackened Chicken

DAIRY-FREE, GLUTEN-FREE, NUT-FREE, SOY-FREE

Serves 4
Prep time: 20 minutes

Cook time: 20 minutes

Cast-iron skillets have a beloved place in American cooks' kitchens. Extremely versatile, they can be used both in the oven and on the stovetop. Here, the skillet blackens chicken to a perfect crisp without losing the juices and seasonings. Naturally nonstick and durable, cast-iron skillets may also give you a nutritional boost by adding a bit of iron to your food.

2 (5-ounce) bone-less, skinless chicken breasts

½ teaspoon paprika

Juice of 1 lemon

½ cup water

2 teaspoons Blackened Rub (page 149)

1 tablespoon olive or avocado oil

1. In a small bowl, massage the chicken all over with the paprika. Add the lemon juice and water and mix. Set aside to marinate for 15 minutes.
2. Remove the chicken from the marinade and shake off the excess liquid.
3. Coat the chicken all over with the blackened rub.
4. Heat a large cast-iron skillet over medium heat. Pour in the olive oil. Add the chicken and cook for 5 to 7 minutes on each side, or until cooked through.
5. Remove the chicken from the heat and let rest for 5 minutes.
6. Divide each breast into two portions.

Prep Tip:

Be sure to space your chicken evenly, as it helps ensure uniform cooking.

Per Serving (½ breast): Calories: 95; Total fat: 4g; Saturated fat: 1g; Sodium: 40mg; Total carbohydrates: 0g; Sugar: 0g; Fiber: 0g; Net carbohydrates: 0g; Protein: 13g

Blackened Rub

Makes ~½ cup

Prep time: 5 minutes

2 tablespoons smoked paprika

2 tablespoons onion powder

2 tablespoons garlic powder

1 tablespoon sweet paprika

1 teaspoon freshly ground black pepper

1 teaspoon dried dill

½ teaspoon ground mustard

¼ teaspoon celery seeds

In an airtight container, mix the smoked paprika, onion powder, garlic powder, sweet paprika, pepper, dill, mustard, and celery seeds.

Storage Tip:

Store for up to 3 months in an airtight container in a cool, dry, and dark place.

Per Serving (1 tablespoon): Calories: 23; Total fat: 1g; Saturated fat: 0g; Sodium: 3mg; Total carbohydrates: 5g; Sugar: 1g; Fiber: 1g; Net carbohydrates: 4g; Protein: 1g

Turkey Meat Loaf

DAIRY-FREE, NUT-FREE, SOY-FREE

Serves 6

Cook time: 1 hour

Prep time: 15 minutes, plus 10 minutes to stand

Meat loaf is often at the top of the list of comfort foods. This recipe cuts way down on the fat by substituting ground turkey for ground beef. Prep and refrigerate this dish the night before, and you'll have dinner for the next evening meal ready to cook and eat. For an additional nutritional punch, experiment by adding grated zucchini or chopped shiitake mushrooms to the mix.

Nonstick cooking spray

1 tablespoon extra-virgin olive oil

1 onion, chopped

3 garlic cloves, minced

1½ pounds ground turkey

½ cup whole wheat bread crumbs

1 large egg

1 teaspoon kosher salt

½ teaspoon freshly ground black pepper

¼ cup ketchup

1. Preheat the oven to 350°F. Lightly coat an 8-by-4-inch loaf pan with cooking spray. Set aside.
2. In a small skillet over medium heat, heat the olive oil.
3. Add the onion and garlic, and sauté for 3 to 5 minutes, until the onion is softened. Remove from the heat, transfer to a large bowl, and let cool for about 5 minutes.
4. Once cooled, add the ground turkey, bread crumbs, egg, salt, and pepper. Mix well to combine. Press the mixture into the prepared loaf pan and spread the ketchup over the top of the loaf. Bake for 50 to 55 minutes, until the internal temperature measures 165°F on an instant-read thermometer.
5. Remove from the oven and let stand for about 10 minutes before slicing into 6 pieces and serving.

Prep Tip:

If you can't find whole wheat bread crumbs at the grocery store, make your own! Save the ends of bread in the freezer in a bag, and when you need them, let them thaw until you can break them into pieces and process in a food processor into crumbs.

Per Serving: Calories: 187; Total fat: 6g; Saturated fat: 1g; Sodium: 620mg; Total carbohydrates: 7g; Sugar: 3g; Fiber: 1g; Net carbohydrates: 6g; Protein: 28g

Ground Turkey Taco Skillet

30 MINUTES OR LESS, GLUTEN-FREE, NUT-FREE, ONE-POT, SOY-FREE

Serves 4
Prep time: 10 minutes

Cook time: 20 minutes

Using prepared salsa is a simple way to add flavor to ground turkey. This is a delicious Southwestern one-pot meal that's versatile, too. You can use leftovers as taco meat or serve them over a bed of lettuce and other greens for a tasty taco salad. Top with your favorite Southwestern toppings, such as sour cream or diced avocados.

1 tablespoon extra-virgin olive oil

1 pound ground turkey

1 onion, chopped

1 green bell pepper, seeded and chopped

½ teaspoon kosher salt

1 small head cauliflower, grated

1 cup corn kernels

½ cup prepared salsa

¼ cup shredded pepper Jack cheese (optional)

1. In a large nonstick skillet over medium-high heat, heat the olive oil until it shimmers.
2. Add the turkey. Cook, crumbling with a spoon, until browned, about 5 minutes.
3. Add the onion, bell pepper, and salt. Cook, stirring occasionally, until the vegetables soften, 4 to 5 minutes.
4. Add the cauliflower, corn, and salsa. Cook, stirring, until the cauliflower rice softens, about 3 minutes more.
5. Sprinkle with the cheese (if using). Reduce the heat to low, cover, and allow the cheese to melt, 2 or 3 minutes.

Storage Tip:

Refrigerate in a sealed container for up to 3 days or freeze for up to 6 months.

Variation:

Using cauliflower in place of rice makes this a low-carb dinner. If you need a few extra grams of carbs, replace the cauliflower with 1 cup of cooked brown rice. It is estimated that 1 cup of cooked rice has 45 grams of carbs, but check the nutrition facts label to be sure.

Per Serving: Calories: 272; Total fat: 14g; Saturated fat: 3g; Sodium: 550mg; Total carbohydrates: 16g; Sugar: 5g; Fiber: 4g; Net carbohydrates: 12g; Protein: 25g

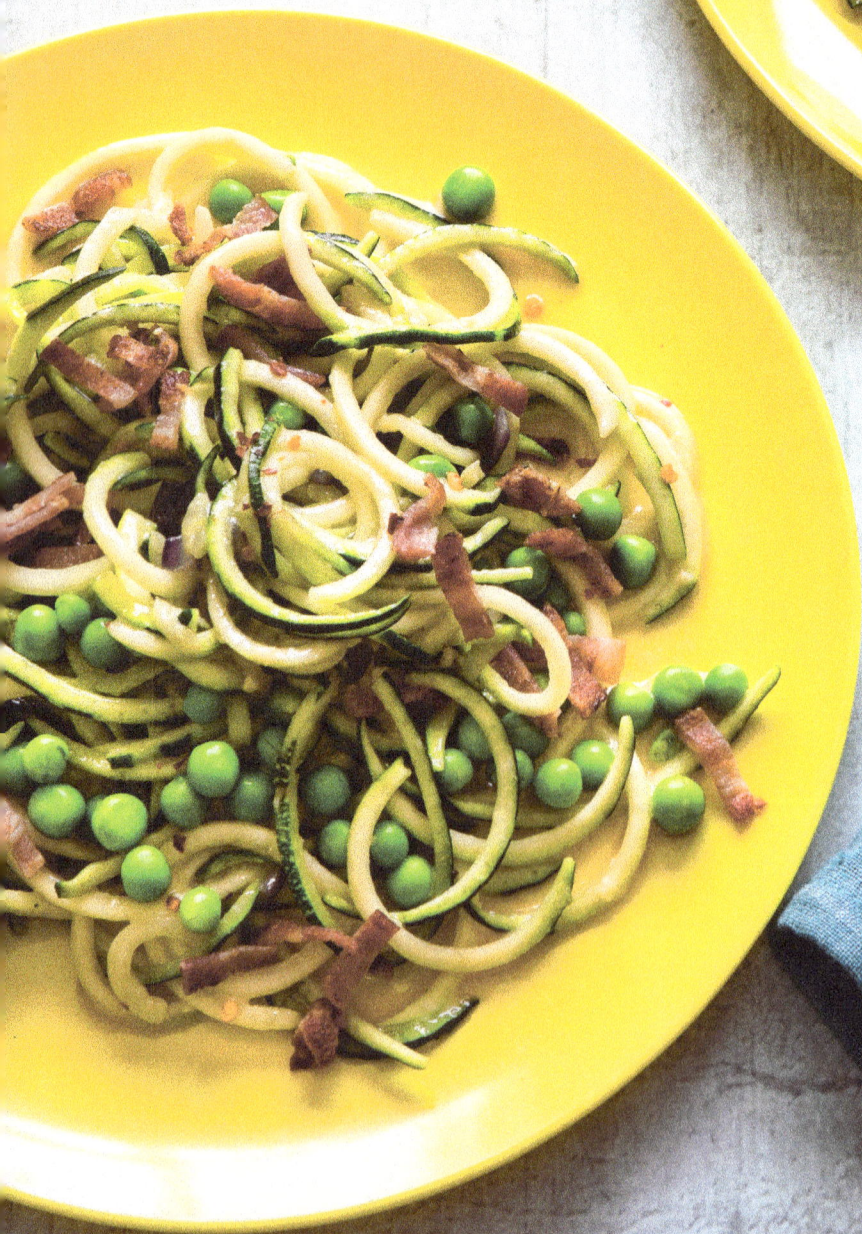

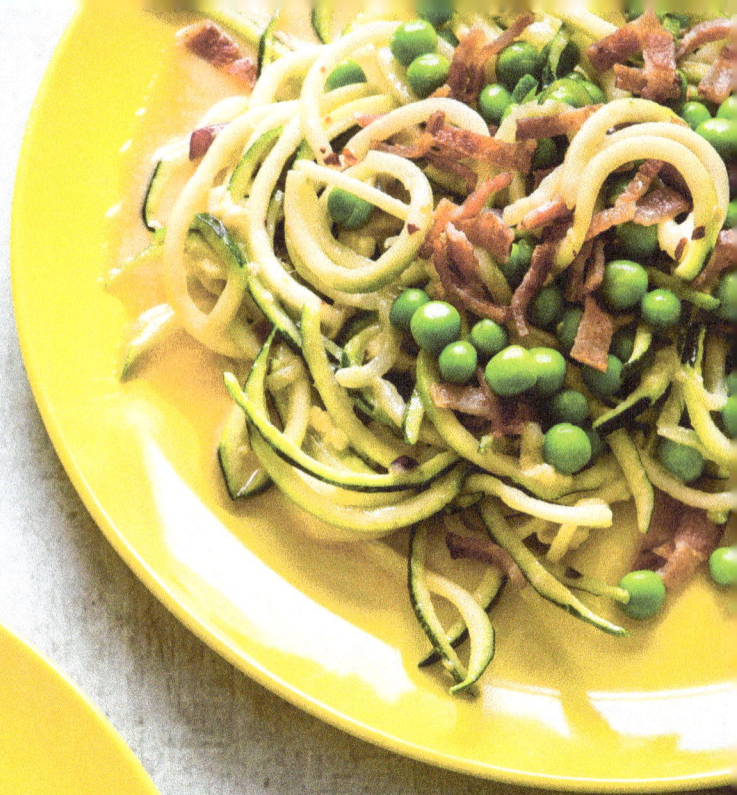

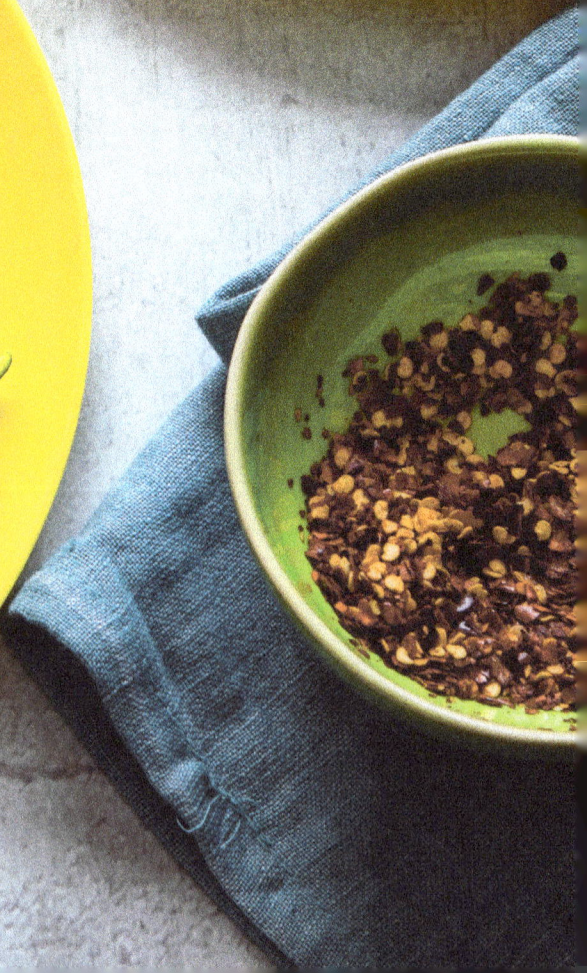

Zoodles Carbonara

GLUTEN-FREE, NUT-FREE, SOY-FREE

Serves 4
Prep time: 10 minutes

Cook time: 25 minutes

Carbonara is a simple bacon-and-egg sauce that is normally served over pasta, but it's delicious on spiralized zucchini, too. It's fast and easy to make.

6 slices turkey bacon, cut into pieces

1 red onion, finely chopped

3 zucchini, cut into noodles

1 cup fresh or thawed frozen peas

½ teaspoon kosher salt

3 garlic cloves, minced

3 large eggs, beaten

Pinch red pepper flakes

¼ cup grated Parmesan cheese (optional, for garnish)

1. In a large skillet over medium-high heat, cook the bacon until browned, about 5 minutes. With a slotted spoon, transfer the bacon to a plate.
2. Add the onion to the bacon fat in the pan and cook, stirring, until soft, 3 to 5 minutes. Add the zucchini, peas, and salt. Cook, stirring, until the zucchini softens, about 3 minutes. Add the garlic and cook, stirring constantly, for 5 minutes.
3. In a small bowl, whisk together the eggs and red pepper flakes. Add to the vegetables.
4. Remove the pan from the stovetop and stir for 3 minutes, allowing the heat of the pan to cook the eggs without setting them.
5. Return the bacon to the pan and stir to mix.
6. Serve topped with Parmesan cheese, if desired.

Storage Tip:

This doesn't keep well. You can refrigerate leftovers, but they won't be as good upon reheating.

Variation:

The peas in this recipe add protein and some carbs. If you need a slightly higher-carb version, you can add more peas. For every additional ½ cup of peas, add 15 grams of carbohydrates.

Per Serving: Calories: 176; Total fat: 8g; Saturated fat: 2g; Sodium: 616mg; Total carbohydrates: 14g; Sugar: 7g; Fiber: 4g; Net carbohydrates: 10g; Protein: 13g

Cioppino (Seafood Stew)

30 MINUTES OR LESS, DAIRY-FREE, NUT-FREE, ONE-POT, SOY-FREE

Serves 4
Prep time: 10 minutes

Cook time: 20 minutes

Cioppino is an Italian American stew that combines seafood and tomatoes. There are many versions, some of which involve using more than one type of fish or shellfish or adding wine. This version is superfast and easy to make, with just a few ingredients and little prep time, but still robust in flavor.

- 1 tablespoon extra-virgin olive oil
- 1 medium onion, chopped
- 1 medium green bell pepper, seeded and chopped
- 1 teaspoon minced garlic
- 1 (28-ounce) can reduced-sodium diced tomatoes
- ½ teaspoon dried basil
- 4 (5-ounce) white-fish fillets, cut into 1-inch chunks

Optional topping
1 (8-ounce) package garlic croutons, divided

1. In a stockpot over medium heat, heat the olive oil until it shimmers. Add the onion, bell pepper, and garlic and sauté until tender, 3 to 5 minutes.
2. Add the tomatoes with their juices and the basil and mix thoroughly. Add the fish, lower the heat, and heat until the fish is cooked, 10 to 15 minutes.
3. Divide the stew into 4 serving bowls. Scatter 2 ounces of optional croutons on top of each bowl, if using.

Storage Tip:

Stew containing seafood should be refrigerated promptly after serving. Refrigerate in an airtight container for up to 5 days or freeze for up to 3 months. Thaw in the refrigerator overnight and reheat in the microwave or on the stovetop.

Per Serving: Calories: 185; Total fat: 5g; Saturated fat: 1g; Sodium: 532mg; Total carbohydrates: 11g; Sugar: 7g; Fiber: 4g; Net carbohydrates: 7g; Protein: 25g

Shrimp and Veggie Skillet

30 MINUTES OR LESS, DAIRY-FREE, GLUTEN-FREE, NUT-FREE, ONE-POT, SOY-FREE

Serves 4
Prep time: 20 minutes

Cook time: 10 minutes

Shrimp is the star of this dish. It's a healthy protein that provides vitamin B_{12}, iron, zinc, copper, and omega-3 fatty acids. For extra veggies and fewer carbs, this dish is served over riced cauliflower instead of rice.

- 1 tablespoon extra-virgin olive oil
- 1 pound raw small shrimp, peeled and deveined (fresh or frozen; no need to thaw)
- ½ cup low-sodium vegetable broth
- 1 medium onion, chopped
- 1 large red bell pepper, seeded and chopped
- 1 large zucchini, diced
- 1 large yellow squash, diced
- 1 large carrot, peeled and sliced
- ½ teaspoon minced garlic
- ½ teaspoon sweet paprika
- 4 cups Cauliflower Rice (see page 213)

1. In a skillet, heat the olive oil over medium heat until it shimmers. Add the shrimp and cook for 1 to 2 minutes per side, until pink.
2. Add the broth, onion, bell pepper, zucchini, squash, carrot, garlic, and paprika and mix well. Cover and cook for 5 to 8 minutes, until all the vegetables are heated through.
3. Serve over warm cauliflower rice.

Per Serving: Calories: 197; Total fat: 5g; Saturated fat: 1g; Sodium: 398mg; Total carbohydrates: 19g; Sugar: 9g; Fiber: 6g; Net carbohydrates: 13g; Protein: 21g

Baked Parmesan-Crusted Halibut

30 MINUTES OR LESS, NUT-FREE, SOY-FREE

Serves 4
Prep time: 10 minutes

Cook time: 15 minutes

For those who don't like the strong flavor of most oily ocean fish, halibut is for you. The mild, sweet taste of this whitefish brings omega-3s to the table—and halibut is also an excellent source of protein, potassium, and niacin. The crunchy panko bread crumb coating is seasoned with Parmesan cheese and garlic powder and enhances the halibut's flavor. To achieve a crispy crust on both top and bottom, place the fish on a rack atop your baking sheet.

Nonstick cooking spray
½ cup whole wheat panko bread crumbs
¼ cup shredded Parmesan cheese

1 tablespoon minced fresh parsley leaves
½ teaspoon garlic powder

½ teaspoon kosher salt
¼ teaspoon freshly ground black pepper
Juice of ½ lemon

1 tablespoon extra-virgin olive oil
1 pound halibut fillet

1. Preheat the oven to 450°F. Place a rack on a baking sheet, and lightly spray with cooking spray.
2. On a large plate, combine the panko bread crumbs, Parmesan, parsley, garlic powder, salt, and pepper, and mix well.
3. Pour the lemon juice and olive oil over both sides of the halibut and press the halibut into the coating mixture. Flip the fish and press the coating onto the other side.
4. Transfer the fish to the prepared rack on the baking sheet, and lightly spray the top of the fish with cooking spray. Bake for 12 to 15 minutes, until the fish flakes easily with a fork, and serve.

Variation:

Panko bread crumbs are Japanese-style bread crumbs that are lighter and airier than the Italian variety. If you can't find whole wheat panko near you, it is readily available online.

Per Serving: Calories: 194; Total fat: 8g; Saturated fat: 2g; Sodium: 432mg; Total carbohydrates: 5g; Sugar: 0g; Fiber: 1g; Net carbohydrates: 4g; Protein: 26g

Salmon and Veggie Bake

DAIRY-FREE, GLUTEN-FREE, NUT-FREE, SOY-FREE

Serves 4
Prep time: 15 minutes

Cook time: 20 to 22 minutes

When you're short on time and dinner ideas, this protein-packed recipe is your ticket. You can save even more time by chopping the veggies the night before and preparing a healthy side such as brown rice, herbed roasted potatoes, or sautéed Brussels sprouts. Cleanup is a snap if you line the pan with parchment paper.

- 1 medium zucchini, chopped into 1-inch pieces
- 1 red bell pepper, seeded and chopped into 1-inch pieces
- 1 medium onion, cut into wedges
- 2 tablespoons extra-virgin olive oil, divided
- ½ teaspoon kosher salt, divided
- ½ teaspoon freshly ground black pepper, divided
- 3 garlic cloves, minced
- 2 teaspoons Dijon mustard
- Juice of 1 lemon
- 1 pound salmon fillet, cut into 4 pieces

1. Preheat the oven to 425°F.
2. In a large bowl, combine the zucchini, red bell pepper, and onion. Add 1 tablespoon of olive oil and toss to coat. Season with ¼ teaspoon each of salt and pepper. Spread the vegetables on a large baking sheet in a single layer and bake for 10 minutes.
3. In the same bowl, whisk the remaining 1 tablespoon of olive oil with the garlic, mustard, lemon juice, and remaining ¼ teaspoon each of salt and pepper. Divide the mixture among the salmon fillets and rub it into the flesh.
4. Once the vegetables have cooked for 10 minutes, nestle the salmon fillets on top of them. Bake for 10 to 12 minutes more, until the salmon flakes easily with a fork and the vegetables are tender. Serve the salmon with the vegetables.

Prep Tip:

Zucchini and bell peppers are great for this recipe because they are quick cooking but still take a little longer than the salmon to cook through. Be sure to get them into the oven and prepare the seasonings for the salmon while they are cooking to make the best use of time.

Per Serving: Calories: 247; Total fat: 14g; Saturated fat: 2g; Sodium: 379mg; Total carbohydrates: 8g; Sugar: 4g; Fiber: 2g; Net carbohydrates: 6g; Protein: 24g

Easy Tuna Patties

30 MINUTES OR LESS, DAIRY-FREE, NUT-FREE, SOY-FREE

Serves 4
Prep time: 5 minutes, plus 10 minutes to chill

Cook time: 10 minutes

By themselves, these patties are low in carbs, even with the inclusion of whole wheat bread crumbs. You can enjoy them with a knife and fork, or if you have a few carbs to spare, put them on slices of whole-grain toast as an open-faced sandwich.

1 pound canned tuna, drained

1 cup whole wheat bread crumbs

2 large eggs, beaten

½ onion, grated

1 tablespoon chopped fresh dill, plus more for garnish

Juice and grated zest of 1 lemon, plus lemon wedges for serving

1 tablespoon extra-virgin olive oil

Chopped chives, for garnish

½ cup low-fat tartar sauce, for serving

1. In a large bowl, combine the tuna, bread crumbs, eggs, onion, dill, and lemon juice and zest. Form the mixture into 4 patties and chill for 10 minutes.
2. In a large nonstick skillet over medium-high heat, heat the olive oil until it shimmers. Add the patties and cook until browned on both sides, 4 to 5 minutes per side.
3. Serve topped with the tartar sauce.

Storage Tip:

Refrigerate leftovers in a sealed container for up to 3 days.

Variation:

Making this an open-faced sandwich with one slice of whole wheat bread adds an estimated 15 grams of carbs. You can also serve this with a simple side salad of non-starchy veggies and a low-sugar vinaigrette for a complete meal.

Per Serving: Calories: 264; Total fat: 9g; Saturated fat: 2g; Sodium: 653mg; Total carbohydrates: 18g; Sugar: 5g; Fiber: 2g; Net carbohydrates: 16g; Protein: 28g

Shrimp Peri-Peri

30 MINUTES OR LESS, DAIRY-FREE, GLUTEN-FREE, NUT-FREE, SOY-FREE

Serves 4
Prep time: 10 minutes

Cook time: 15 minutes

Peri-peri sauce (also called piri-piri) is a spicy South African–inspired sauce you can enjoy on just about any type of protein, from shrimp to beef. This shrimp cooks quickly under the broiler, and the sauce is fragrant and flavorful without overpowering the inherently sweet, briny flavor of the shrimp.

1 recipe Peri-Peri Sauce (page 223)	1 pound large shrimp, shelled and deveined	2 tablespoons extra-virgin olive oil	Kosher salt

1. Preheat the oven broiler on high.
2. In a small pot, bring the peri-peri sauce to a simmer.
3. Meanwhile, place the cleaned shrimp on a rimmed baking sheet, deveined-side down. Brush with the olive oil and sprinkle with salt.
4. Broil until opaque, about 5 minutes. Serve with the sauce on the side for dipping or spooned over the top of the shrimp.

Storage Tip:

Cook this on demand. Store cooked shrimp separately from sauce for up to 3 days in the refrigerator.

Variation:

Serve this dish with a ¼-cup serving of cooked quinoa on the side (9 grams of carbs, 1 gram of fiber) and some steamed non-starchy veggies, such as broccoli.

Per Serving: Calories: 279; Total fat: 16g; Saturated fat: 2g; Sodium: 464mg; Total carbohydrates: 10g; Sugar: 2g; Fiber: 3g; Net carbohydrates: 7g; Protein: 24g

Cod with Mango Salsa

30 MINUTES OR LESS, DAIRY-FREE, GLUTEN-FREE, NUT-FREE, SOY-FREE

Serves 4
Prep time: 10 minutes

Cook time: 10 minutes

Cod is a mild-flavored, low-fat, white-fleshed fish; you can replace it with whatever whitefish is available in your area. Be sure to carefully remove any pin bones using a pair of needle-nose tweezers to pull the bones away from the flesh. The salsa complements the sweet flesh of the cod perfectly. Serve with vegetables and whole grains to create a balanced meal with the right number of carbs.

1 pound cod, cut into 4 fillets, pin bones removed

2 tablespoons extra-virgin olive oil

¾ teaspoon kosher salt, divided

1 mango, pitted, peeled, and cut into cubes

¼ cup chopped cilantro

½ red onion, finely chopped

1 jalapeño pepper, seeded and finely chopped

1 garlic clove, minced

Juice of 1 lime

1. Preheat the oven broiler on high.
2. On a rimmed baking sheet, brush the cod with the olive oil and season with ½ teaspoon of the salt. Broil until the fish is opaque, 5 to 10 minutes.
3. Meanwhile, in a small bowl, combine the mango, cilantro, onion, jalapeño, garlic, lime juice, and remaining ¼ teaspoon of salt.
4. Serve the cod with the salsa spooned over the top.

Storage Tip:

Cook this on demand. Store the cooked cod separately from the salsa for up to 3 days in the refrigerator.

Variation:

Reduce carbs by replacing the mango with 1 large chopped tomato. Serve this dish with a side salad and vinaigrette or a steamed non-starchy veggie. For more carbs, add steamed brown rice.

Per Serving: Calories: 197; Total fat: 8g; Saturated fat: 1g; Sodium: 432mg; Total carbohydrates: 13g; Sugar: 10g; Fiber: 2g; Net carbohydrates: 11g; Protein: 21g

Teriyaki Salmon

30 MINUTES OR LESS, DAIRY-FREE, NUT-FREE

Serves 4
Prep time: 5 minutes

Cook time: 5 minutes

Teriyaki has a sweet, salty flavor that pairs nicely with the sweet flavor of salmon. To make this gluten-free, you can use gluten-free tamari. If you can't find rice vinegar, regular white vinegar is an acceptable substitute.

⅓ cup pineapple juice
⅓ cup reduced-sodium soy sauce
¼ cup water

2 tablespoons rice vinegar
1 tablespoon honey
1 garlic clove, minced

1 teaspoon peeled and grated fresh ginger
Pinch red pepper flakes

1 pound salmon fillet, cut into 4 pieces

1. Preheat the oven broiler on high.
2. In a small bowl, whisk together the pineapple juice, soy sauce, water, vinegar, honey, garlic, ginger, and red pepper flakes.
3. Place the salmon pieces flesh-side down in the mixture for 5 minutes.
4. Place the salmon on a rimmed baking sheet, flesh-side up. Gently brush with any leftover sauce.
5. Broil until the salmon is opaque, 3 to 5 minutes.

Storage Tip:

Refrigerate in a sealed container for up to 3 days.

Variation:

This is a very-low-carb recipe, even with the honey and pineapple juice. You can increase the carbs by serving it with a side of steamed veggies.

Per Serving: Calories: 202; Total fat: 7g; Saturated fat: 1g; Sodium: 752mg; Total carbohydrates: 9g; Sugar: 6g; Fiber: <1g; Net carbohydrates: 8g; Protein: 24g

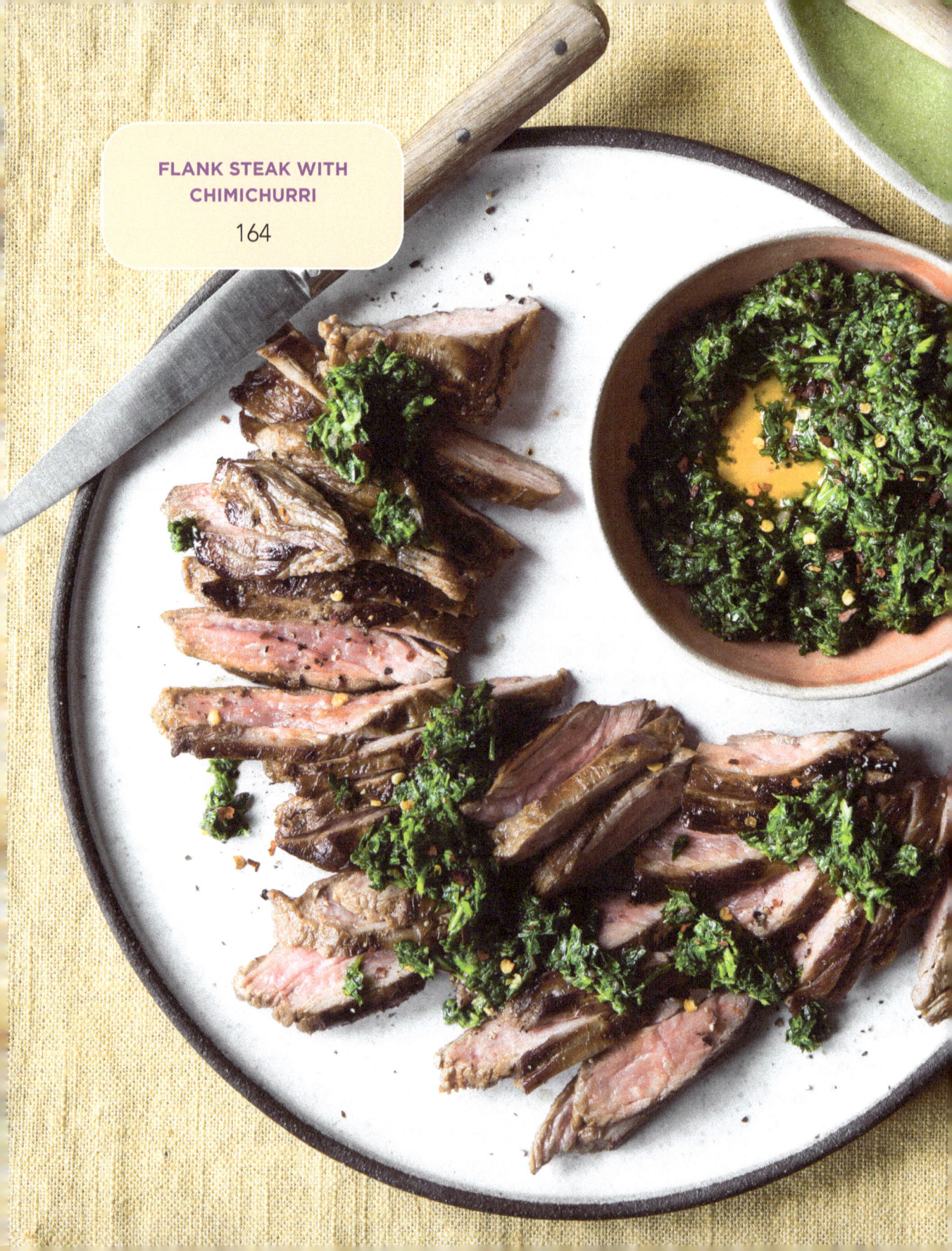

FLANK STEAK WITH CHIMICHURRI

164

7

BEEF AND PORK

Flank Steak with Chimichurri

30 MINUTES OR LESS, DAIRY-FREE, GLUTEN-FREE, NUT-FREE, SOY-FREE

Serves 4
Prep time: 15 minutes

Cook time: 10 minutes

A lean, nutritious, boneless cut with lots of intense beef flavor, flank steak has more protein per ounce (about 8 grams) than other steak cuts like porterhouse or rib eye. Remember to cut across the grain when serving, which yields a more tender piece of meat.

For the chimichurri

¼ cup packed fresh parsley leaves

¼ cup packed fresh cilantro leaves

¼ cup chopped red onion

1 garlic clove, peeled

2 tablespoons extra-virgin olive oil

2 tablespoons water

1 tablespoon apple cider vinegar

¼ teaspoon kosher salt

Freshly ground black pepper

Red pepper flakes

For the flank steak

1 pound flank steak, trimmed

1 teaspoon kosher salt

½ teaspoon garlic powder

Freshly ground black pepper

To make the chimichurri

1. In a food processor, combine the parsley, cilantro, onion, garlic, olive oil, water, vinegar, and salt. Pulse a few times until just combined. Season with black pepper and red pepper flakes and set aside.

To make the flank steak

2. Season both sides of the steak with the salt, garlic powder, and some black pepper.
3. Heat a large cast-iron skillet over high heat.
4. Add the steak to the hot pan, and cook for 3 to 5 minutes per side, flipping once, until medium-rare. Transfer to a cutting board and let rest for 5 minutes. Cut into thin strips across the grain and serve topped with the chimichurri.

Per Serving: Calories: 263; Total fat: 17g; Saturated fat: 1g; Sodium: 732mg; Total carbohydrates: 1g; Sugar: 1g; Fiber: 0g; Net carbohydrates: 1g; Protein: 25g

Pot Roast with Vegetables

DAIRY-FREE, GLUTEN-FREE, NUT-FREE, SOY-FREE

Serves 4
Prep time: 15 minutes

Cook time: 1 hour 5 minutes

Making lower-cost meat cuts tender and moist is a snap with the Dutch oven. This recipe uses often-overlooked winter vegetables such as rutabaga and parsnips. Because you're cooking a whole two-pound cut of meat, you'll have leftovers for lunch the next day!

- 1 tablespoon avocado oil
- 1 (2-pound) eye of round roast
- 1 (4-ounce) can sliced mushrooms, drained
- 1 medium onion, chopped
- 4 carrots, cut into ½-inch pieces
- 2 parsnips, cut into ½-inch pieces
- 1 small rutabaga, peeled and cut into 1-inch chunks
- ½ teaspoon freshly ground black pepper
- 1 bay leaf
- 1½ cups water

1. In a Dutch oven over high heat, heat the avocado oil until it shimmers. Add the roast and brown on all sides, about 5 minutes.
2. Lower the heat to medium. Add the remaining ingredients and stir to combine.
3. Cover the pot and simmer for about 1 hour, until the meat and vegetables are fork-tender.

Prep Tip:

When serving meat, especially tougher cuts, remember to slice across the grain (perpendicular to the muscle fibers). This makes the meat easier to chew, because some of the work of breaking down the muscle fibers is already done.

Per Serving (6 ounces cooked beef plus ¼ veggies): Calories: 415; Total fat: 11g; Saturated fat: 3g; Sodium: 122mg; Total carbohydrates: 25g; Sugar: 10g; Fiber: 7g; Net carbohydrates: 18g; Protein: 53g

Steak Fajitas

30 MINUTES OR LESS, NUT-FREE, SOY-FREE

Serves 4
Prep time: 10 minutes

Cook time: 15 minutes

Fajitas are usually made using skirt steak, but this version with round steak makes for tender meat in less time. Round steak comes from the rear leg of the cow—top round and eye of round are more tender than bottom round. This recipe lets everyone in the family personalize their fajita with their very own toppings. Get creative and don't feel limited by the list here!

2 tablespoons avocado oil

12 ounces round steak, thinly sliced

1 teaspoon minced garlic

½ teaspoon chili powder

½ teaspoon ground cumin

¼ teaspoon freshly ground black pepper

1 tablespoon freshly squeezed lime or lemon juice

1 small onion, sliced

1 small green bell pepper, seeded and sliced

8 (6-inch) cauliflower, coconut, or corn tortillas

Toppings, as desired: diced fresh tomatoes, shredded lettuce, salsa, chopped avocado, shredded cheese

1. In a Dutch oven over medium heat, heat the avocado oil until it shimmers. Add the steak and brown on both sides, 3 to 5 minutes. Season with the garlic, chili powder, cumin, black pepper, and lime juice.
2. Add the onion and bell pepper to the pot. Cover and simmer for 5 to 10 minutes, until the meat is tender.
3. Serve the steak mixture in warm tortillas. Top as desired.

Per Serving: Calories: 323; Total fat: 13g; Saturated fat: 3g; Sodium: 375mg; Total carbohydrates: 28g; Sugar: 2g; Fiber: 4g; Net carbohydrates: 24g; Protein: 22g

One-Pot Beef and Veggie Lasagna

NUT-FREE, ONE-POT, SOY-FREE

Serves 6
Prep time: 5 minutes

Cook time: 40 minutes

Lasagna may not be a regular meal for you because it takes time to cook the noodles and create all the layers, but this one-pot version doesn't require much time or effort. All the flavors of lasagna you love—tomato sauce, oregano, cheeses, and ground beef, plus a vegetable surprise—are in this dish without all the work. To make this lasagna meatless, substitute vegan "beef" crumbles from the freezer section in the supermarket. They are protein-packed, without the fat and cholesterol of beef, and are always ready in your freezer.

1 pound 95% lean ground beef

1 medium onion, chopped

1 (24-ounce) jar marinara sauce

1 (8-ounce) container fat-free cottage cheese

8 ounces no-boil lasagna noodles, broken into 3-inch pieces

1 large zucchini, spiralized

1 cup shredded part-skim mozzarella cheese

1 teaspoon dried oregano

1. Preheat the oven to 350°F.
2. In a Dutch oven over medium-high heat, brown the ground beef for about 5 minutes. Drain all excess grease. Add the onion and cook until tender, about 3 minutes.
3. Stir in the marinara sauce. Add the cottage cheese and mix well.
4. Drop in the lasagna noodle pieces and stir to submerge them.
5. Top with the zucchini, mozzarella, and oregano.
6. Cover and bake for 20 to 25 minutes, until the mixture is bubbly. Remove the cover and cook for 2 to 3 more minutes more, until the cheese browns slightly.

Prep Tip:

You can buy ready-made spiralized zucchini (zoodles) packaged in the produce section at the supermarket. Or you can use a carrot peeler to get long, thin slices, then stack them up and cut them lengthwise.

Per Serving: Calories: 354; Total fat: 8g; Saturated fat: 3g; Sodium: 308mg; Total carbohydrates: 41g; Sugar: 8g; Fiber: 4g; Net carbohydrates: 37g; Protein: 32g

Slow-Cooked Traditional Beef Stew

DAIRY-FREE, NUT-FREE, ONE-POT, SOY-FREE

Serves 4
Prep time: 15 minutes

Cook time: 3 hours, 15 minutes

Beef stew is usually a winter dish, but slow cookers don't heat up the kitchen the way a stove does, so this may become a summer favorite. This is a classic combination for beef stew, but you can customize it with your own vegetables. Good options are mixed vegetables, leafy greens, summer or winter squash, sweet potatoes, and root vegetables.

- 1 tablespoon olive or avocado oil
- 1 pound stewing beef chunks
- 2 tablespoons all-purpose flour
- ½ teaspoon freshly ground black pepper
- 1 (6-ounce) can low-sodium tomato paste
- 1 (28-ounce) can low-sodium diced tomatoes
- 3 cups low-sodium beef broth
- 1 tablespoon Worcestershire sauce
- 2 celery stalks, chopped
- 1 large onion, chopped
- 3 large carrots, chopped
- 1 medium potato, scrubbed and cut into ½-inch pieces
- 1 bay leaf

1. In a slow cooker on high, heat the olive oil. Add the beef and sauté for 8 to 10 minutes, until it starts to brown. Add the flour and pepper and stir to coat.
2. Add the tomato paste, tomatoes with their juices, broth, Worcestershire sauce, celery, onion, carrots, potato, and bay leaf. Stir to combine, cover, and bring the mixture to a boil.
3. Reduce the heat to low and simmer for 3 hours, until the beef is tender. Remove the bay leaf before serving.

Variation:

Try using lean ground turkey instead of stew beef in this recipe. Ground turkey offers a different texture than the stew beef—more like sloppy Joes.

Per Serving: Calories: 368; Total fat: 11g; Saturated fat: 0g; Sodium: 305mg; Total carbohydrates: 37g; Sugar: 17g; Fiber: 7g; Net carbohydrates: 30g; Protein: 31g

Miso Skirt Steak

30 MINUTES OR LESS, DAIRY-FREE, NUT-FREE

Serves 4
Prep time: 20 minutes

Cook time: 5 to 10 minutes

While meat shouldn't be the primary source of your calories or macronutrients, know that you can still enjoy steak on occasion. Here, it is flavorfully prepared with miso and soy.

3 tablespoons yellow miso

1 tablespoon reduced-sodium soy sauce or tamari

½ tablespoon sesame oil

2 tablespoons chile-garlic sauce

1½ pounds skirt steak, patted dry

3 tablespoons rice vinegar

1 tablespoon vegetable oil, divided

1. In a medium bowl, whisk together the miso, soy sauce, sesame oil, and chile-garlic sauce. Put 1 tablespoon of the sauce in a separate small bowl and set aside. Place the steak in the bowl with the remaining sauce and marinate it at room temperature for 10 to 15 minutes.
2. Stir the vinegar and ½ tablespoon of vegetable oil into the reserved sauce and set aside.
3. Remove the steak from the bowl and pat it dry.
4. Heat the remaining ½ tablespoon of vegetable oil in a large skillet over medium-high heat, add the steak, and cook without disturbing it. Cook for 2 to 3 minutes, until brown. Flip the steak and repeat with the other side (bring to 125°F internal temperature for medium rare and 135°F for medium). Transfer the steak to a plate, tent it with foil, and allow it to rest for 5 to 10 minutes.
5. Serve with the sauce on the side.

Variation:

Keep the meal simple and serve the steak with salad greens, cooked whole grains, Cauliflower Rice (page 213), or a mixture of all three options.

Per Serving: Calories: 206; Total fat: 11g; Saturated fat: 3g; Sodium: 450mg; Total carbohydrates: 4g; Sugar: 1g; Fiber: 1g; Net carbohydrates: 3g; Protein: 20g

Lebanese-Inspired Beef Kebabs with Pickled Onions

30 MINUTES OR LESS, GLUTEN-FREE, DAIRY-FREE, NUT FREE, SOY-FREE

Serves 4
Prep time: 20 minutes

Cook time: 10 minutes

These spiced beef kebabs are both flavorful and healthy. Using a variety of spices can truly eliminate the need for added salt, which is a bonus for your heart. Serve these tender kebabs with curried rice or throw an ear of corn on the grill while you're cooking the beef.

1 red bell pepper, seeded and chopped

½ onion, coarsely chopped

2 garlic cloves, coarsely chopped

1 pound 95% lean ground beef

1½ teaspoons ground cumin

1½ teaspoons sumac (optional)

1½ teaspoons red pepper flakes

1 teaspoon kosher salt

Freshly ground black pepper

1 tablespoon ice-cold water

1 teaspoon vegetable oil

Pickled Red Onions (page 171)

8 (12-inch) metal skewers (or wooden skewers soaked in warm water for 10 to 30 minutes)

1. Place the red bell pepper, onion, and garlic in a food processor and pulse until they're very finely chopped but not pureed. Set aside in a bowl, draining off any excess liquid.

2. Put the beef, processed vegetables, cumin, sumac (if using), red pepper flakes, salt, and a pinch of black pepper into the bowl of a stand mixer with the paddle attached. Work on medium speed until the mix starts sticking to the sides of the bowl, about a minute. Add the ice-cold water and mix for another 5 minutes, until you have a sticky mass. Chill the meat mixture in the freezer for a few minutes or in the refrigerator for at least 30 minutes (or overnight).

3. Divide the meat mixture into 8 balls. With a small bowl of cold water beside you, wet your hands and form the kebab mixture around the skewers, distributing it evenly until you have kofta about 9 inches long and 2 inches thick. Smooth out any holes or tears, then place them on a greaseproof paper–lined baking sheet.

4. Grease a grill pan with the vegetable oil and place it over high heat. Grill the kofta until charred on the outside and just cooked through, 8 to 10 minutes. Put the grilled kebabs directly on top of the pickled red onions, so the juices drip onto the onions, and serve.

Per Serving: Calories: 199; Total fat: 7g; Saturated fat: 3g; Sodium: 369mg; Total carbohydrates: 7g; Sugar: 3g; Fiber: 1g; Net carbohydrates: 6g; Protein: 25g

Pickled Red Onions

Makes 1½ cups   **Prep time:** 3 minutes

1 red onion, thinly sliced

1 cup cider vinegar

1 tablespoon whole
  black peppercorns
  (optional)

In a small bowl, combine the red onion with the vinegar and black peppercorns. Allow the onions to marinate for at least 15 minutes and up to 1 hour at room temperature. Serve immediately or store in the refrigerator in an airtight container for up to 1 week.

Per Serving (¼ cup): Calories: 16; Total fat: 0g; Saturated fat: 0g; Sodium: 3mg; Total carbohydrates: 2g; Sugar: 1g; Fiber: 0g; Protein: 0g

Creole Braised Sirloin

DAIRY-FREE, GLUTEN-FREE, NUT-FREE, ONE-POT, SOY-FREE

Serves 4
Prep time: 15 minutes

Cook time: 40 minutes

Like cast-iron skillets, Dutch ovens have been in the United States since at least the 1700s. Truly versatile, they can be used over an open flame as easily as in an oven. In this recipe, it's used to make a mouthwatering, lean, Creole-seasoned steak.

- 1 pound beef round sirloin tip, cut into 4 strips
- ¼ teaspoon freshly ground black pepper
- 2 cups Chicken Broth (page 225) or store-bought low-sodium chicken broth, divided
- 1 medium onion, chopped
- 1 celery stalk, coarsely chopped
- 1 medium green bell pepper, seeded and coarsely chopped
- 2 garlic cloves, minced
- 4 medium tomatoes, coarsely chopped
- 1 bunch mustard greens including stems, coarsely chopped
- 1 tablespoon Creole seasoning (see tip, page 176)
- ¼ teaspoon red pepper flakes
- 2 bay leaves

1. Preheat the oven to 450°F.
2. Massage the beef all over with the black pepper.
3. In a Dutch oven, bring 1 cup of broth to a simmer over medium heat.
4. Add the onion, celery, bell pepper, and garlic and cook, stirring often, for 5 minutes, or until the vegetables are softened.
5. Add the tomatoes, mustard greens, Creole seasoning, and red pepper flakes and cook for 3 to 5 minutes, or until the greens are wilted.
6. Add the bay leaves, beef, and remaining 1 cup of broth.
7. Cover the pot, transfer to the oven, and cook for 30 minutes, or until the juices run clear when you pierce the beef.
8. Remove the beef from the oven and let rest for 5 to 7 minutes. Discard the bay leaves.
9. Thinly slice the beef and serve.

Per Serving (4 ounces sirloin, ½ cup vegetables each): Calories: 202; Total fat: 5g; Saturated fat: 2g; Sodium: 129mg; Total carbohydrates: 14g; Sugar: 7g; Fiber: 5g; Net carbohydrates: 9g; Protein: 28g

Loaded Cottage Pie

DAIRY-FREE, NUT-FREE, SOY-FREE

Serves 6
Prep time: 15 minutes

Cook time: 1 hour

In this decadent cottage pie, you'll find a dish both nutritious and delicious. The vegetable filling, a mix of collard greens, tomatoes, and carrots, provides an array of phytonutrients that benefit your overall health, helping to reduce oxidative stress and systemic inflammation. Finishing this pie with potatoes forms a perfect crunchy topping.

3 large russet potatoes, peeled and halved

2 tablespoons extra-virgin olive oil, divided

1 small onion, chopped

1 bunch collard greens, stemmed and thinly sliced

2 carrots, peeled and chopped

2 medium tomatoes, chopped

1 garlic clove, minced

1 pound 95% lean ground beef

½ cup Chicken Broth (page 225) or store-bought low-sodium chicken broth

1 teaspoon Worcestershire sauce

1 teaspoon celery seeds

1 teaspoon smoked paprika

½ teaspoon dried chives

½ teaspoon ground mustard

½ teaspoon cayenne pepper

1. Preheat the oven to 400°F.
2. Bring a large pot of water to a boil.
3. Add the potatoes and boil for 15 to 20 minutes, or until fork-tender.
4. Transfer the potatoes to a large bowl and mash with 1 tablespoon of olive oil.
5. In a large cast-iron skillet, heat the remaining 1 tablespoon of olive oil.
6. Add the onion, collard greens, carrots, tomatoes, and garlic and sauté, stirring often, for 7 to 10 minutes, or until the vegetables are softened.
7. Add the beef, broth, Worcestershire sauce, celery seeds, and smoked paprika.
8. Spread the meat and vegetable mixture evenly onto the bottom of a casserole dish. Sprinkle the chives, ground mustard, and cayenne on top of the mixture. Spread the mashed potatoes evenly over the top.
9. Transfer the casserole dish to the oven, and bake for 30 minutes, or until the top is light golden brown.

Per Serving (¾ cup): Calories: 318; Total Fat: 9g; Saturated fat: 2g; Sodium: 117mg; Total carbohydrates: 39g; Sugar: 4g; Fiber: 5g; Net carbohydrates: 34g; Protein: 22g

Bean and Beef Taco Wraps

30 MINUTES OR LESS, NUT-FREE, ONE-POT, SOY-FREE

Serves 4
Prep time: 10 minutes

Cook time: 15 minutes

These appetizing wraps are sure to please everyone at the table. Use lean ground round beef, which has a lower fat content than ground chuck but still has all the flavor. The fiber in black beans adds bulk while also lowering fat. Whole wheat tortillas are a traditional way of eating these wraps, but you can make them lighter by serving on lettuce leaves. Round out the meal with sliced apples and steamed carrots.

8 ounces 95% lean
  ground beef

½ cup cooked
  black beans

½ cup salsa, divided

1 teaspoon
  onion powder

1 teaspoon
  chili powder

¼ teaspoon
  garlic powder

Freshly ground
  black pepper

4 (8-inch) whole wheat
  flour tortillas

1 cup finely sliced
  lettuce, divided

1. In a large skillet over medium-high heat, cook the beef for about 7 minutes, until browned and cooked through. Drain.
2. Add the black beans, ¼ cup of salsa, and the onion powder, chili powder, and garlic powder. Season with pepper and stir to combine. Bring the mixture to a boil, reduce the heat to low, and simmer for 5 minutes.
3. Into each tortilla, spoon one-quarter of the meat mixture, ¼ cup of lettuce, and 1 tablespoon of the remaining salsa, and serve.

Prep Tip:

The meat mixture can be made up to 3 days in advance. When ready to serve, simply reheat and fill the tortillas, top with lettuce, and enjoy.

Per Serving: Calories: 246; Total fat: 7g; Saturated fat: 3g; Sodium: 467mg; Total carbohydrates: 27g; Sugar: 3g; Fiber: 7g; Net carbohydrates: 20g; Protein: 23g

Mushroom and Beef Burgers

30 MINUTES OR LESS, DAIRY-FREE, NUT-FREE, SOY-FREE

Serves 4
Prep time: 10 minutes

Cook time: 20 minutes

A good burger is something we all crave now and then. To keep fat and calories under control, use ground round beef and form a four-ounce patty (about the size and thickness of the palm of your hand). The mushrooms keep it lean without losing any of the meaty flavor you expect. Grilling or broiling is also an acceptable lean-cooking method for these.

8 ounces cremini mushrooms

1 tablespoon extra-virgin olive oil

1 onion, finely chopped

3 garlic cloves, minced

8 ounces 95% lean ground beef

½ teaspoon kosher salt

¼ teaspoon freshly ground black pepper

4 whole wheat hamburger buns

Ketchup, for serving

Mustard, for serving

Lettuce leaves, for serving

1. In a food processer, pulse the mushrooms a few times until coarsely ground.
2. In a large skillet over medium-high heat, heat the olive oil.
3. Add the ground mushrooms, onion, and garlic, and sauté for 8 to 10 minutes, until the vegetables soften and the liquid evaporates. Remove from the pan, and cool completely.
4. In a large bowl, combine the ground beef, cooled mushroom mixture, salt, and pepper. Mix well. Form the meat mixture into 4 patties.
5. Return the skillet to medium-high heat. Add the patties, and cook for 3 to 5 minutes per side, until cooked to your desired level of doneness.
6. Serve on the buns, topped with ketchup, mustard, and lettuce leaves.

Per Serving: Calories: 261; Total fat: 8g; Saturated fat: 2g; Sodium: 417mg; Total carbohydrates: 31g; Sugar: 9g; Fiber: 5g; Net carbohydrates: 26g; Protein: 18g

Red Beans and Rice with Pulled Pork

DAIRY-FREE, GLUTEN-FREE, NUT-FREE, ONE-POT, SOY-FREE

Serves 4   **Cook time:** 1 hour
Prep time: 10 minutes

A Southern and Creole favorite, this recipe gets a protein punch from the pulled pork. Traditionally, leftover pork from Sunday's meal was added to the beans for a filling start to the week. Together, the pulled pork, rice, and beans make a well-balanced, satisfying meal.

15 ounces ready-to-eat pulled pork, without barbecue sauce

2 (16-ounce) cans kidney beans, drained and rinsed

1 medium onion, chopped

1 cup chopped celery

4 cups low-sodium chicken broth

1 bay leaf

1 teaspoon freshly ground black pepper

1 teaspoon salt-free Creole seasoning blend (see tip, below)

1½ cups cooked brown rice

1. In a large stockpot, combine the pulled pork, beans, onion, celery, broth, bay leaf, pepper, and Creole seasoning. Bring the mixture to a boil over medium heat.
2. Lower the heat, cover, and simmer, stirring occasionally, for 1 hour, or until the mixture begins to thicken.
3. Remove the bay leaf.
4. Divide the rice between four bowls, top with the pulled pork and beans, and serve.

Prep Tip:

You can make your own sodium-free Creole seasoning blend by mixing equal amounts of freshly ground black pepper, garlic powder, sweet paprika, cayenne pepper, dried oregano, and dried thyme.

Per Serving: Calories: 412; Total fat: 5g; Saturated fat: 2g; Sodium: 393mg; Total carbohydrates: 56g; Sugar: 2g; Fiber: 10g; Net carbohydrates: 46g; Protein: 35g

Mushroom Pork Chops with Potatoes and Onions

GLUTEN-FREE, NUT-FREE, SOY-FREE

Serves 4
Prep time: 15 minutes

Cook time: 35 minutes

This recipe will quickly become a family favorite. The pork stays juicy and flavorful in the Dutch oven as the potatoes slowly cook in the gravy. Layering the ingredients makes this dish simple to prepare but fancy to serve.

1 tablespoon extra-virgin olive or avocado oil

4 (4-ounce) boneless pork chops

1 (10½-ounce) can 98% fat-free condensed cream of mushroom soup

1 cup unsweetened almond milk

4 medium baking potatoes, scrubbed and cut into ¼-inch slices

1 large onion, sliced

Freshly ground black pepper

2 tablespoons chopped fresh parsley

1. Preheat the oven to 350°F.
2. In a Dutch oven over medium heat, heat the olive oil until it shimmers. Add the pork chops and brown them on both sides, about 5 minutes. Transfer the pork chops to a plate.
3. Pour the soup and almond milk into the Dutch oven and mix until smooth. Layer the potatoes, onion, and pork chops in the soup mixture. Sprinkle pepper on top.
4. Cover and bake until the potatoes are fork-tender, about 30 minutes.
5. Garnish with ½ tablespoon of parsley per serving.

Variation:

Baking potatoes work well in this recipe thanks to their texture, but you can use russet, Yukon Gold, or red-skinned potatoes, too. Leaving the skin on the potatoes adds extra nutrients, including fiber.

Per Serving: Calories: 398; Total fat: 9g; Saturated fat: 3g; Sodium: 543mg; Total carbohydrates: 47g; Sugar: 3g; Fiber: 5g; Net carbohydrates: 42g; Protein: 30g

Bean and Pork Stew

DAIRY-FREE, GLUTEN-FREE, NUT-FREE, SOY-FREE

Serves 4
Prep time: 10 minutes

Cook time: 25 minutes

This hearty stew provides a great balance of protein and carbohydrates. Beans are the main protein, and pork is a flavor add-in. As with most recipes that use canned beans, feel free to mix it up and use whatever beans you have on hand.

1 tablespoon extra-virgin olive oil

2 (4-ounce) bone-less, trimmed pork chops, cut into ¼-inch chunks

1 large red onion, chopped

1 tablespoon minced garlic

2 large carrots, thinly sliced

2 (15-ounce) cans great northern beans, rinsed and drained

1 (12-ounce) package frozen cut green beans (no need to thaw)

4 cups low-sodium vegetable broth

½ teaspoon dried thyme

1 teaspoon honey mustard

1. In a Dutch oven over medium heat, heat the olive oil until it shimmers. Add the pork and sauté until just cooked through, about 5 minutes. Transfer the pork to a plate with a slotted spoon and set aside. Add the onion and garlic to the skillet and sauté until tender, about 3 minutes.
2. Add the carrots, beans, green beans, broth, reserved pork, thyme, and honey mustard to the pot and stir well. Bring to a boil, then reduce the heat and simmer for 15 to 20 minutes, until the mixture is hot.

Prep Tip:

You can also use canned or frozen sliced carrots; because they're already cooked, the stew will cook even faster.

Per Serving: Calories: 327; Total fat: 6g; Saturated fat: 1g; Sodium: 178mg; Total carbohydrates: 42g; Sugar: 5g; Fiber: 13g; Net carbohydrates: 29g; Protein: 26g

Pork and Apple Skillet

30 MINUTES OR LESS, DAIRY-FREE, GLUTEN-FREE, NUT-FREE, ONE-POT

Serves 4
Prep time: 10 minutes

Cook time: 20 minutes

Pork and apples are a great combination, particularly in the fall, when apples are in season. Choose a tart-sweet apple, such as Honeycrisp, Granny Smith, or Cripps Pink. Save time by using coleslaw mix instead of shredding a head of cabbage.

1 tablespoon extra-virgin olive oil

1 pound boneless, trimmed pork chops, cut into ¼-inch slices

1 red onion, thinly sliced

2 apples, peeled, cored, and thinly sliced

2 cups shredded cabbage

1 teaspoon dried thyme

2 garlic cloves, minced

¼ cup apple cider vinegar

1 tablespoon Dijon mustard

½ teaspoon kosher salt

⅛ teaspoon freshly ground black pepper

1. In a large skillet over medium-high heat, heat the olive oil and cook the pork chops until browned, turning halfway through, about 12 minutes. Transfer the pork to a plate.
2. Add the onion, apples, cabbage, and thyme to the fat in the skillet. Cook, stirring occasionally, until the vegetables are soft, about 5 minutes.
3. Add the garlic and cook, stirring constantly, for 5 minutes.
4. Return the pork chops to the skillet.
5. In a small bowl, whisk together the vinegar, mustard, salt, and pepper. Add to the skillet. Bring to a simmer. Cook, stirring, until the sauce thickens, about 2 minutes.

Storage Tip:

Refrigerate in a sealed container for up to 3 days or freeze for up to 6 months.

Variation:

This dish is delicious served with sautéed Swiss chard, which is a green leafy vegetable that adds few carbs and is an excellent source of calcium.

Per Serving: Calories: 242; Total fat: 8g; Saturated fat: 3g; Sodium: 251mg; Total carbohydrates: 17g; Sugar: 10g; Fiber: 3g; Net carbohydrates: 14g; Protein: 20g

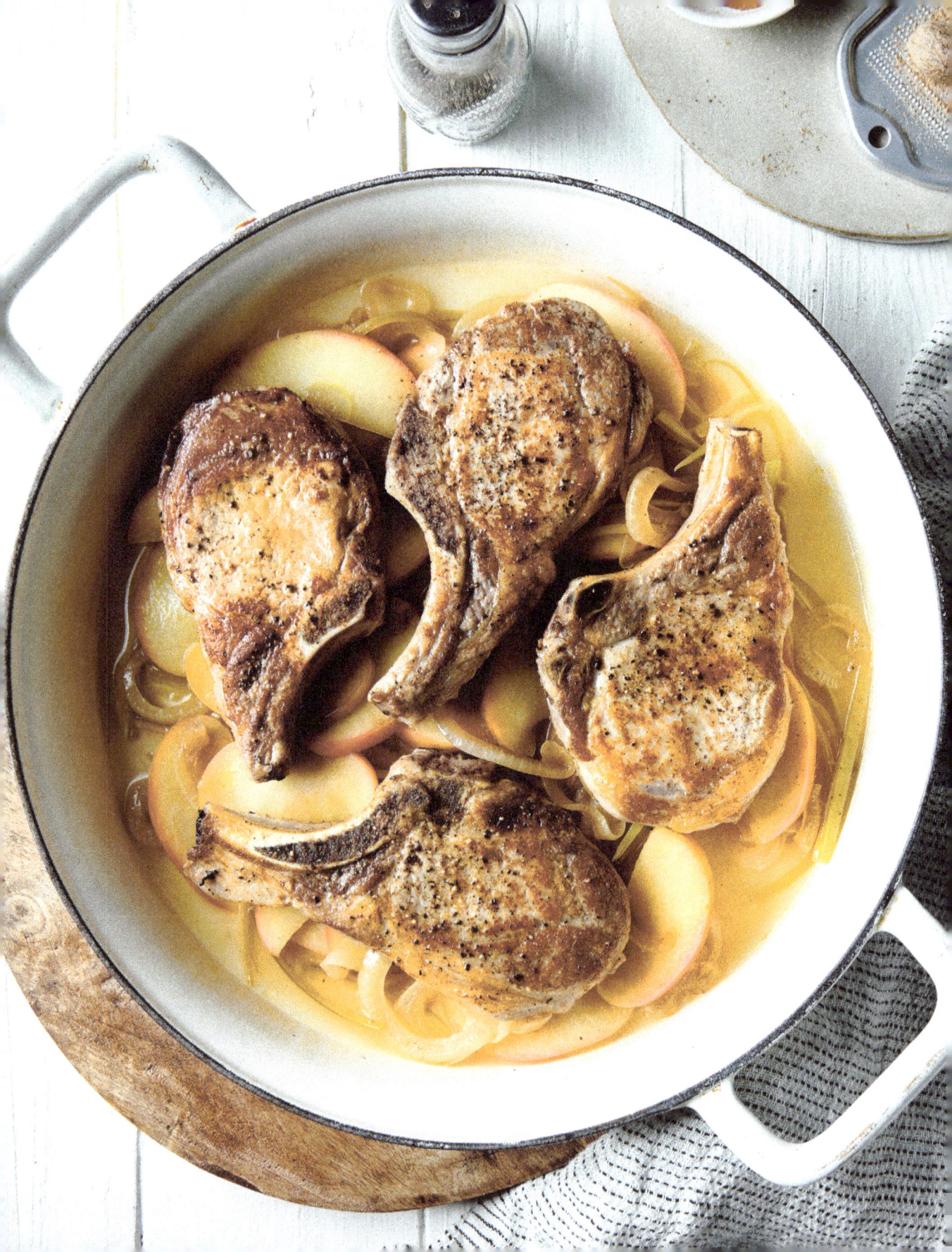

Dutch Oven Apple Pork Chops

DAIRY-FREE, GLUTEN-FREE, NUT-FREE, SOY-FREE

Serves 4
Prep time: 20 minutes

Cook time: 20 minutes

By nature, pork chops are a lean cut of meat. To keep your chop juicy and flavorful, this recipe calls for generously seasoning the meat and taking care not to dry it out through overcooking. The lively combination of the sweet apple and mild celery, in concert with the earthy pork, will make your taste buds dance.

4 bone-in pork loin chops, trimmed

¼ cup apple cider vinegar

1 teaspoon freshly ground black pepper

1 teaspoon ground cinnamon

1 teaspoon ground nutmeg

½ cup Chicken Broth (page 225) or store-bought low-sodium chicken broth

3 celery stalks, cut into matchsticks

1 large apple, thinly sliced

½ cup chopped onion

1. Put the pork chops on a rimmed baking sheet. Season both sides of the pork chops with the vinegar, pepper, cinnamon, and nutmeg.
2. In a Dutch oven, bring the broth to a simmer over medium heat.
3. Add the pork chops and cook for 3 minutes, or until the exterior is browned. Transfer to a plate.
4. Add the celery, apple, and onion to the pot, making a bed.
5. Place the pork chops on top and cover. Cook for 10 to 15 minutes, taking care not to overcook.
6. Serve each pork chop with a generous spoonful of apple, celery, and onion on the side.

Per Serving: Calories: 208; Total fat: 5g; Saturated fat: 2g; Sodium: 436mg; Total carbohydrates: 10g; Sugar: 6g; Fiber: 3g; Net carbohydrates: 7g; Protein: 30g

Pulled Pork Loin

DAIRY-FREE, NUT-FREE, SOY-FREE

Serves 8
Prep time: 30 minutes

Cook time: 3 hours

Marinades, like the one used in this pork loin preparation, can add deep flavor and nutrition. In this pulled pork classic, dietary fiber–rich onions and their culinary cousin garlic bring lots of punchy flavor to the marinade. Using steam heat to cook the vegetables and spices along with the meat produces a juicy, savory platter certain to please you and any guests.

2 pounds boneless pork sirloin roast

1 tablespoon ground mustard seeds

1 tablespoon olive oil

½ cup Chicken Broth (page 225) or store-bought low-sodium chicken broth

1 medium zucchini, grated

1 medium carrot, grated

1 medium onion, chopped

2 medium tomatoes, chopped

½ cup tomato paste

½ cup apple cider vinegar

2 tablespoons Pepper Sauce (page 222)

1 tablespoon Worcestershire sauce

2 garlic cloves, minced

1 teaspoon Baltimore-Style Seasoning (page 183)

1. Preheat the oven to 300°F. Massage the pork all over with the mustard seeds and set aside for 20 minutes.
2. In a large Dutch oven or skillet, heat the olive oil over medium-high heat. Brown the pork on all sides, about 7 minutes in total. If using a skillet, transfer the pork to a large ovenproof casserole dish. Add the broth, zucchini, carrot, onion, tomatoes, tomato paste, vinegar, pepper sauce, Worcestershire sauce, garlic, and seasoning.
3. Cover and cook in the oven for 2½ to 3 hours until the meat is very tender, adding more liquid if too dry.
4. Transfer the pork to a clean, flat surface, and shred the meat using two forks.
5. Return the pork to the Dutch oven or casserole dish and mix into the juices.

Storage Tip:

This dish can be refrigerated for up to 5 days in an airtight container.

Per Serving (4 ounces): Calories: 282; Total fat: 19g; Saturated fat: 2g; Sodium: 127mg; Total carbohydrates: 8g; Sugar: 5g; Fiber: 2g; Net carbohydrates: 6g; Protein: 21g

Baltimore-Style Seasoning

30 MINUTES OR LESS, GLUTEN-FREE, NUT-FREE, ONE-POT, SOY-FREE, VEGAN

Makes about ½ cup

Prep time: 10 minutes

3 tablespoons
sweet paprika

2 tablespoons
celery seeds

1 tablespoon mus-
tard seeds

2 teaspoons freshly
ground black pepper

1½ teaspoons
cayenne pepper

1 teaspoon red
pepper flakes

½ teaspoon
ground nutmeg

½ teaspoon ground
cinnamon

½ teaspoon
ground ginger

¼ teaspoon
ground cloves

In an airtight container, combine the paprika, celery seeds, mustard seeds, black pepper, cayenne, red pepper flakes, nutmeg, cinnamon, ginger, and cloves.

Storage Tip:

Store for up to 3 months in an airtight container in a cool, dry, and dark place.

Per Serving (1 tablespoon): Calories: 27; Total fat: 2g; Saturated fat: 0g; Sodium: 4mg; Total carbohydrates: 4g; Sugar: 1g; Fiber: 2g; Net carbohydrates: 2g; Protein: 1g

Herb-Crusted Pork Tenderloin

DAIRY-FREE, NUT-FREE, SOY-FREE

Serves 4
Prep time: 10 minutes

Cook time: 25 minutes

This lean cut of pork is widely available and very easy and quick to cook. The moist meat gets a flavor boost from the herbs and spices, while the whole wheat panko bread crumb coating adds crunchiness. Serve it with brown rice and roasted veggies, such as asparagus and red bell peppers.

1 teaspoon ground mustard

1 teaspoon kosher salt

½ teaspoon freshly ground black pepper

1 (1-pound) pork tenderloin, trimmed

2 tablespoons extra-virgin olive oil, divided

1 cup whole wheat panko bread crumbs

2 teaspoons minced fresh thyme

1 garlic clove, minced

½ teaspoon ground cumin

1 tablespoon Dijon mustard

1. Preheat the oven to 425°F.
2. In a small bowl, stir together the ground mustard, salt, and pepper, and rub the spices over the tenderloin.
3. In a large cast-iron skillet or other oven-safe skillet over medium-high heat, heat 1 tablespoon of olive oil.
4. Add the pork and sear on all sides, about 2 minutes per side, until browned.
5. Meanwhile, in a small bowl, stir together the bread crumbs, thyme, garlic, cumin, and remaining 1 tablespoon of olive oil.
6. Spread the Dijon mustard on the top of the tenderloin and press the bread crumb mixture into it. Transfer the skillet to the oven and bake for 12 to 15 minutes, until the internal temperature measures 140°F on an instant-read thermometer and the juices run clear.
7. Let rest for 5 minutes before slicing and serving.

Per Serving: Calories: 301; Total fat: 13g; Saturated fat: 2g; Sodium: 220mg; Total carbohydrates: 21g; Sugar: 1g; Fiber: 2g; Net carbohydrates: 19g; Protein: 26g

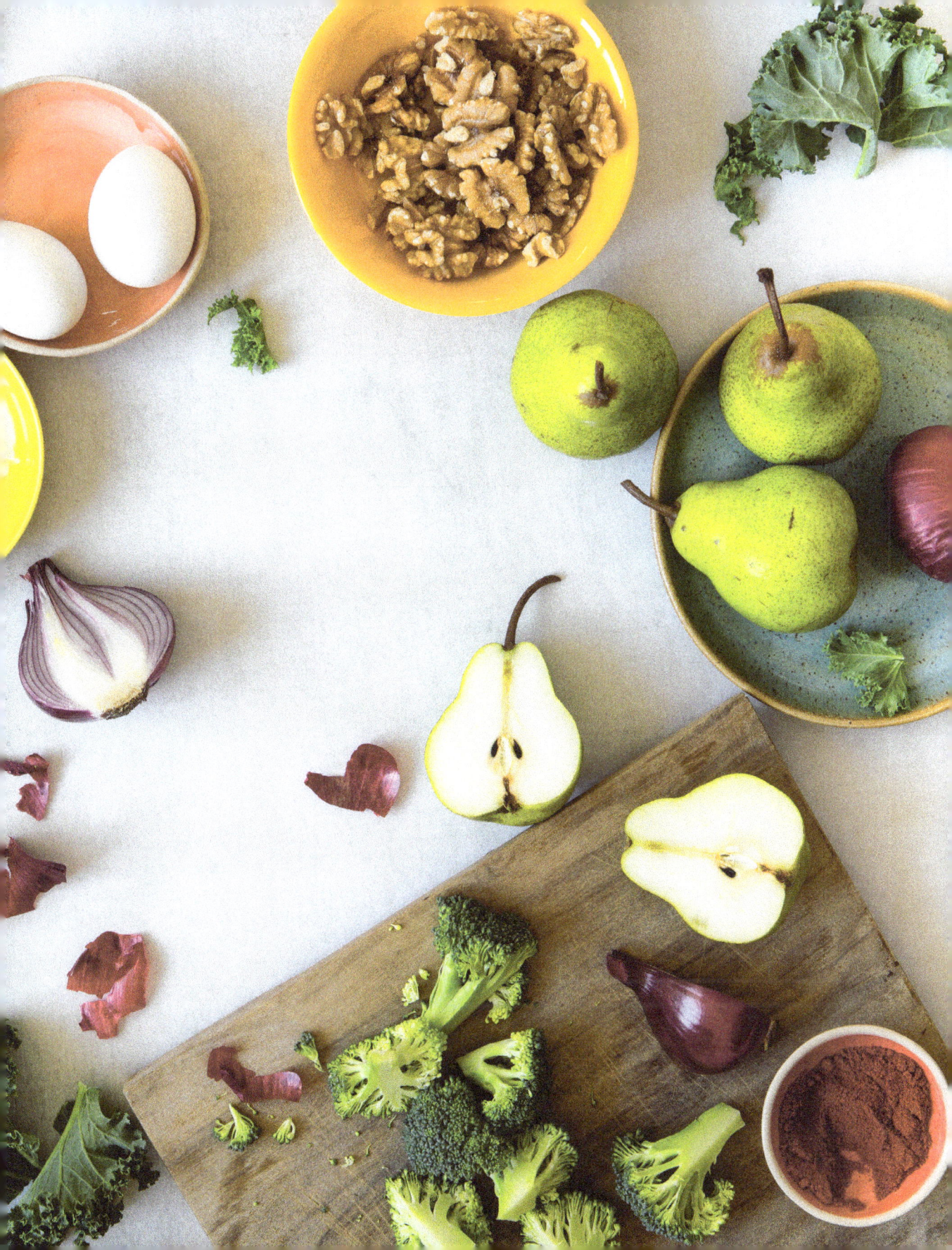

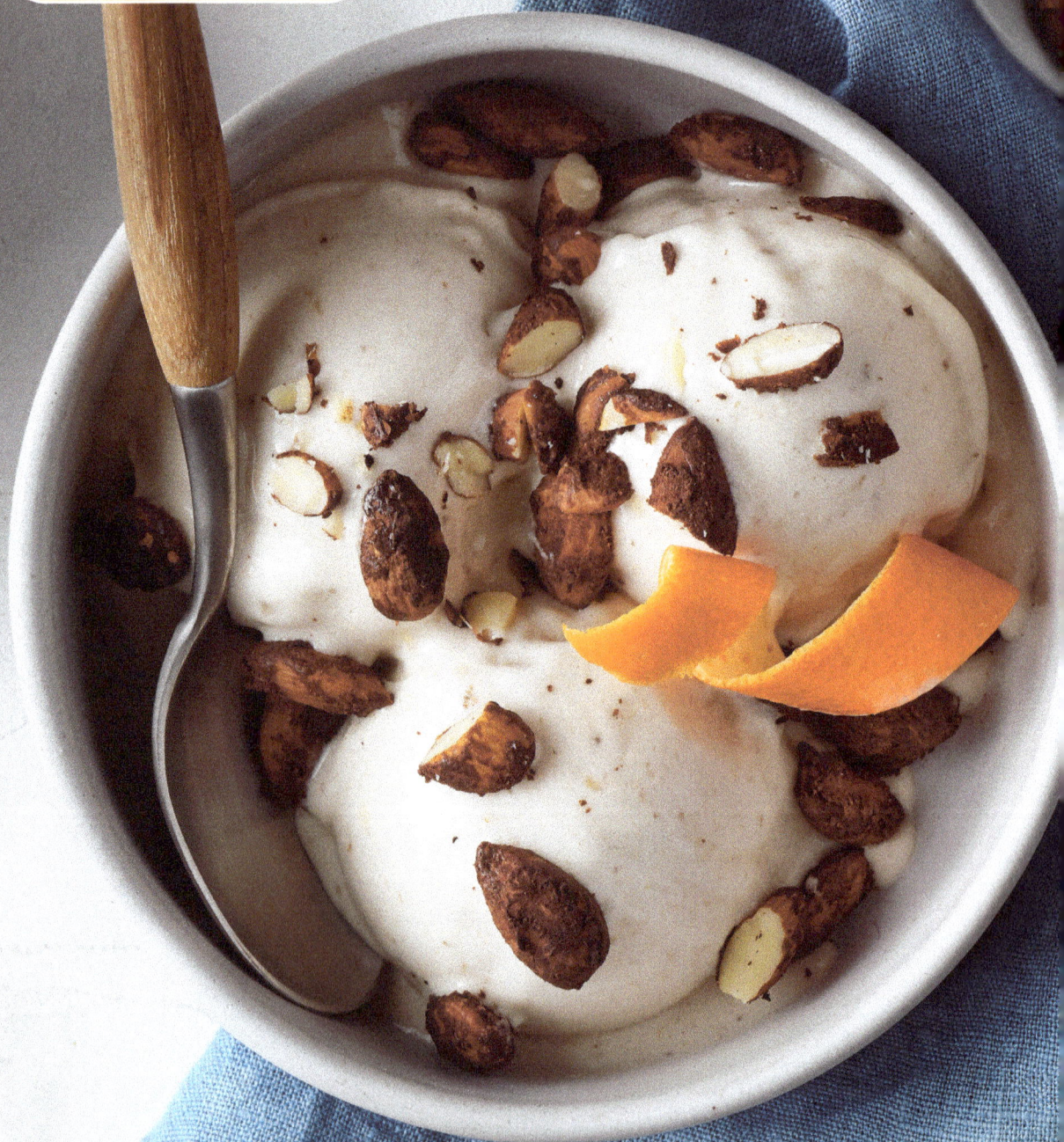

BANANA N'ICE CREAM WITH COCOA NUTS

194

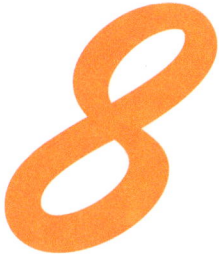

8

DESSERTS

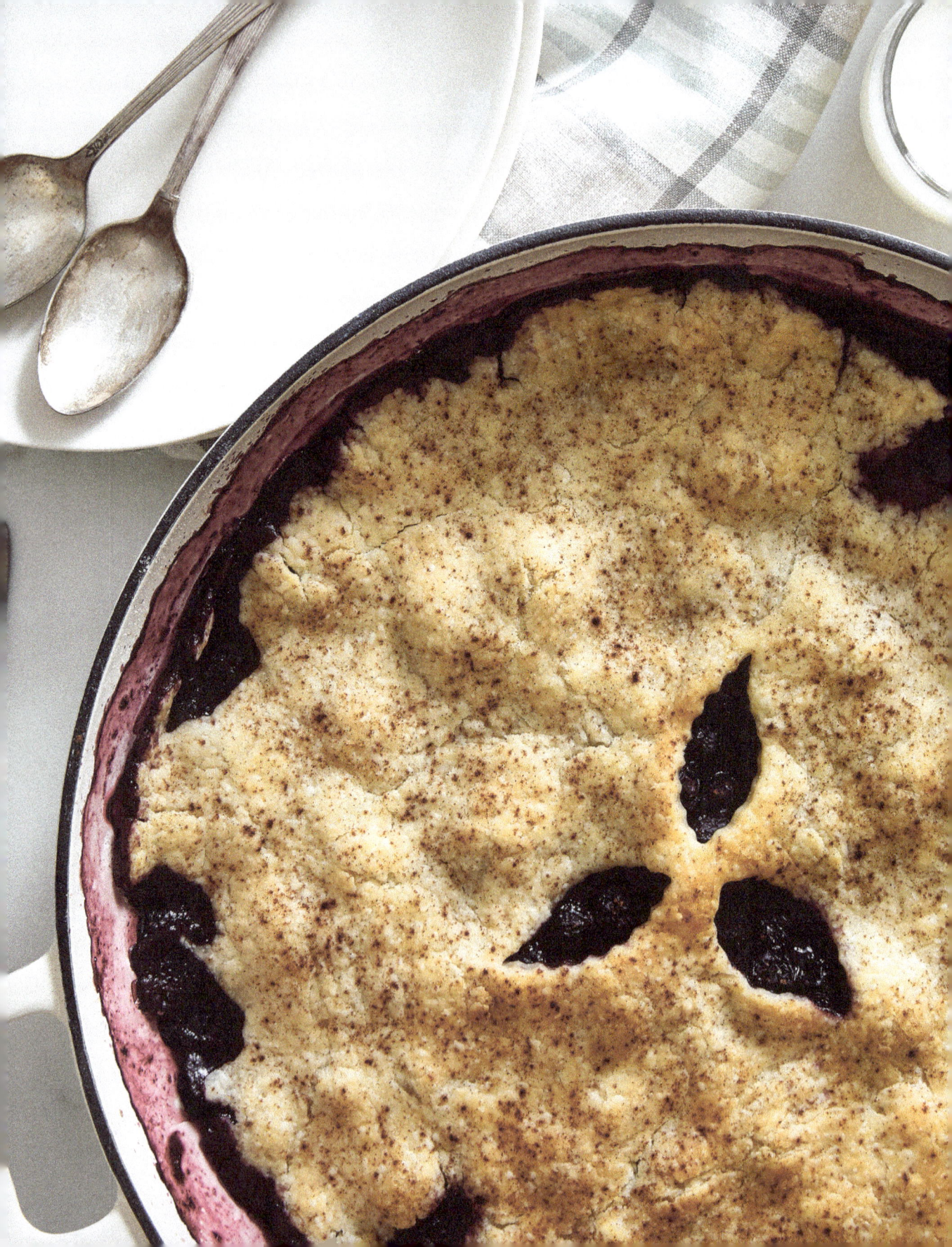

Skillet Berry Cobbler

NUT-FREE, ONE-POT, SOY-FREE, VEGETARIAN

Serves 4
Prep time: 10 minutes

Cook time: 30 to 35 minutes

This is cobbler at its best! Like a fruit pie but without a bottom crust, this cobbler is juicy and bubbling with natural sweetness. You can use a variety of different berries, either frozen or fresh-picked. Add a small amount of zero-calorie sweetener if you want a sweeter cobbler.

1½ cups raspberries, blueberries, strawberries, and/or blackberries (fresh or frozen)

1 to 2 packets zero-calorie sweetener, such as stevia or Truvia (optional)

2 tablespoons freshly squeezed lemon juice

1 premade piecrust

Cinnamon, for garnish (optional)

1. Put an oven-safe skillet in the oven and preheat the oven to 350°F.
2. When the oven comes up to heat, carefully remove the skillet from the oven. In the hot pan, stir together the berries, sweetener (if using), and lemon juice. Cover the berries with the piecrust. Cut 3 slits in the top to allow steam to escape and dust lightly with cinnamon (if using).
3. Bake for 30 to 35 minutes, until the crust is golden brown.

Per Serving: Calories: 194; Total fat: 11g; Saturated fat: 2g; Sodium: 206mg; Total carbohydrates: 22g; Sugar: 4g; Fiber: 2g; Net carbohydrates: 20g; Protein: 2g

Apple-Cranberry Crisp

GLUTEN-FREE, NUT-FREE, SOY-FREE, VEGAN

Serves 6   Cook time: 50 to 55 minutes
Prep time: 30 minutes

Apples are high in fiber, vitamin C, and antioxidants. They help keep your immune system working to prevent illness. Apple skins give your body soluble and insoluble fiber in the form of pectin, so keeping the skin on the apple means you are getting all the nutrition the apple has to offer. The dried cranberries also keep your immune system functioning well, and they're known for having a protective effect against urinary tract infections.

For the topping

1 cup gluten-free
   rolled oats

1 teaspoon ground
   cinnamon

2 tablespoons coconut
   oil, melted

For the crumble

Nonstick cooking spray

5 McIntosh or
   Granny Smith
   apples (unpeeled),
   cored and cut into
   ½-inch slices

¼ cup unsweetened
   dried cranberries

¼ cup unsweetened
   apple juice

1 teaspoon ground
   cinnamon

1. Preheat the oven to 350°F.
2. In a small bowl, combine the oats, cinnamon, and coconut oil using a fork or pastry cutter, until small crumbles form. Set aside.
3. Spray the casserole dish with nonstick cooking spray. Combine the apples, cranberries, apple juice, and cinnamon in the casserole dish and mix well.
4. Sprinkle the topping mixture over the apples.
5. Bake for 50 to 55 minutes, until the dish is bubbly and golden brown.

Prep Tip:

You can use canned apple pie filling in this recipe as a time-saver, but read the label and buy the brand with the least amount of added sugar.

Per Serving: Calories: 198; Total fat: 6g; Saturated fat: 3g; Sodium: 7mg; Total carbohydrates: 36g; Sugar: 19g; Fiber: 6g; Net carbohydrates: 30g; Protein: 3g

Grilled Watermelon with Avocado Mousse

GLUTEN-FREE, NUT-FREE, SOY-FREE, VEGETARIAN

Serves 8
Prep time: 10 minutes

Cook time: 10 minutes

Putting a watermelon on the grill both evolves the flavor and adds a fun presentation twist. Watermelons are 92 percent water, so they are incredibly hydrating, as well as a good source of vitamin C. Pairing the grilled watermelon with a spicy avocado mousse creates a dish with many levels of flavor.

1 small, seedless watermelon, halved and cut into 1-inch rounds

2 ripe avocados, pitted and peeled

½ cup fat-free plain yogurt

¼ teaspoon cayenne pepper

1. On a hot grill, grill the watermelon slices for 2 to 3 minutes on each side, or until you can see the grill marks.
2. To make the avocado mousse, in a blender, combine the avocados, yogurt, and cayenne and process until smooth.
3. To serve, cut each watermelon round in half. Top each with a generous dollop of avocado mousse.

Prep Tip:

If the avocado is not quite ripe, you can wrap it in foil, and bake it in the oven for 10 to 15 minutes to soften it up.

Per Serving (1 full round): Calories: 126; Total fat: 7g; Saturated fat: 1g; Sodium: 14mg; Total carbohydrates: 13g; Sugar: 8g; Fiber: 4g; Net carbohydrates: 9g; Protein: 3g

Watermelon-Lime Granita

GLUTEN-FREE, NUT-FREE, SOY-FREE, VEGAN

Serves 10

Prep time: 15 minutes

Freeze time: 2½ hours

Cool and refreshing, this granita is perfect for the hot days of summer. While this recipe is quick and easy to make, it does require a bit of preplanning for it to taste best. The pureed fruit takes about 2½ hours to freeze and turn into a delicious slush, so make sure you plan ahead if serving this dessert.

1 pound seedless watermelon flesh, cut into 1-inch chunks

2 tablespoons agave syrup

2 tablespoons freshly squeezed lime juice

1. Line a baking sheet with parchment paper. Spread the watermelon chunks in a single layer on the sheet and freeze for at least 20 minutes.
2. Once the chunks are frozen, transfer them to a blender with the agave syrup and lime juice. Blend until liquefied and pour the mixture into a 9-by-13-inch shallow baking dish. Return to the freezer and freeze for 2 hours.
3. Every 30 minutes or so, take a fork and scrape the crystals into a slush consistency.

Storage Tip:

Keep in the freezer for up to 1 month.

Variation:

Surprise your palate and guests by adding a pinch of cayenne or chili powder to make the granita spicy. Substitute another type of citrus for the lime and different kinds of melon to create refreshing variations.

Per Serving: Calories: 27; Total fat: <1g; Saturated fat: 0g; Sodium: 1mg; Total carbohydrates: 7g; Sugar: 5g; Fiber: <1g; Net carbohydrates: 6g; Protein: <1g

Blueberry Chocolate Yogurt Bark

GLUTEN-FREE, SOY-FREE, VEGETARIAN

Serves 15   **Prep time:** 5 minutes, plus 3 hours to set

Bark is a popular treat in many gourmet shops because it looks gorgeous and is fun to eat. Making your own version is incredibly easy, and you don't have to wait for a holiday to enjoy it. Chocolate and blueberries are full of antioxidants and can help boost brain health.

3 cups plain
  Greek yogurt

2 tablespoons honey

2 teaspoons
  vanilla extract

2 cups blueberries

½ cup dark choco-
  late chips

1. Line a baking sheet with parchment paper.
2. In a medium bowl, stir the yogurt, honey, and vanilla until well combined. Spread the yogurt on the baking sheet into a rectangle about 12 by 15 inches.
3. Scatter the blueberries and chocolate chips evenly over the entire surface of the yogurt.
4. Freeze until firm, about 2 ½ to 3 hours. Break the bark into 30 pieces and serve.

Storage Tip:

Freeze the bark in a sealed container for up to 2 weeks.

Variation:

All berries will work for this bark, although you should cut larger berries into ¼-inch pieces. You could ditch the berries altogether and add other fresh fruit. Just be sure to cut the fruit into ¼-inch pieces.

Per Serving: Calories: 86; Total fat: 3g; Saturated fat: 2g; Sodium: 36mg; Total carbohydrates: 11g; Sugar: 9g; Fiber: 1g; Net carbohydrates: 10g; Protein: 3g

Banana N' Ice Cream with Cocoa Nuts

30 MINUTES OR LESS, GLUTEN-FREE, SOY-FREE, VEGAN

Serves 4
Prep time: 10 minutes

Cook time: 12 minutes

If you are in danger of a frozen banana avalanche every time you open the freezer, this is the recipe for you. If your frozen bananas are whole, you will have to give them a rough chop before adding them to the food processor. If you don't have any frozen bananas, slice fresh bananas into small pieces, freeze them for three hours or overnight, then follow the recipe.

For the cocoa nuts

- ¼ cup freshly squeezed orange juice
- 1 tablespoon coconut oil
- 2 teaspoons cocoa powder
- ¼ teaspoon kosher salt
- ¼ teaspoon ground cinnamon
- ¼ teaspoon ground cardamom
- ½ teaspoon grated orange zest
- 1 cup raw almonds

For the banana n'ice cream

- 2 frozen, diced bananas

To make the cocoa nuts

1. Preheat the oven to 350°F. Line a baking sheet with parchment paper.
2. In a small saucepan, bring the orange juice to a boil over medium-high heat, reduce the heat to low, and simmer until the juice is reduced to about 2 tablespoons, 5 to 7 minutes. Add the coconut oil, stir until well combined, and remove from the heat. Whisk in the cocoa powder, salt, cinnamon, cardamom, and zest. Then add the almonds and stir to coat them. Spread the mixture onto the prepared baking sheet.
3. Bake the nuts for 10 to 12 minutes, stirring halfway through, until toasted. Allow to cool, then roughly chop (if you like).

To make the banana n'ice cream

4. Put the frozen bananas in a food processor and pulse. Scrape down the sides, then pulse once more. Continue to do this for several minutes until the texture resembles ice cream. Serve immediately with the cooled nuts.

Storage Tip:

Store the nuts in an airtight container at room temperature for up to 2 weeks.

Variation:

Skip the nuts and only make the banana n'ice cream; that way, you only need one ingredient for a delectable dessert!

Per Serving: Calories: 299; Total fat: 20g; Saturated fat: 3g; Sodium: 79mg; Total carbohydrates: 23g; Sugars: 10g; Fiber: 6g; Net carbohydrates: 17g; Protein: 8g

Superfood Brownie Bites

30 MINUTES OR LESS, GLUTEN-FREE, SOY-FREE, VEGAN

Makes 30 | **Prep time:** 15 minutes

Words like "superfood" get tossed around often. What exactly qualifies an ingredient as a superfood? In this case, it's the combination of nuts, seeds, cacao, and naturally sweet dates, all of which offer benefits to your body. Show up to any party with a platter of these brownie bites and watch them disappear.

1 cup raw nuts (walnuts, pecans, or cashews)

½ cup hulled hemp seeds

⅓ cup raw pepitas

½ cup raw cacao powder

1 cup pitted dates

2 tablespoons coconut oil

1 teaspoon vanilla extract

1. Line a baking sheet with parchment paper.
2. Place the nuts, hemp seeds, and pepitas in a food processor and pulse until the ingredients are a meal consistency. Add the cacao powder, dates, coconut oil, and vanilla and pulse until the mixture holds together if you pinch it with your fingers. The dough should ball up and appear glossy, and not be too sticky and wet. If it doesn't stick together enough to form a dough consistency, add water in drops until the correct consistency is reached. Be careful not to add too much liquid. If you do, add more cacao to balance the texture.
3. Scoop out the brownie bite mixture in 1-tablespoon amounts and roll the mixture into balls. Set the balls on the baking sheet, then chill them in the refrigerator for at least 10 minutes to hold their shape.
4. Transfer the balls to a container with a lid and store in the refrigerator until ready to eat. You could eat these immediately, but they are more likely to crumble.

Storage Tip:

Refrigerate the brownies in an airtight container for 5 to 7 days.

Per Serving (1 bite): Calories: 86; Total fat: 6g; Saturated fat: 1g; Sodium: 2mg; Total carbohydrates: 7g; Sugar: 3g; Fiber: 2g; Net Carbohydrates: 5g; Protein: 3g

Poached Pears

30 MINUTES OR LESS, GLUTEN-FREE, SOY-FREE, VEGAN

Serves 4
Prep time: 10 minutes

Cook time: 20 minutes

Choosing fruit for dessert over sugar-filled pastries, cakes, and pies is a clear choice if you're looking to cut back on carbohydrates and calories, because whole fruit has more fiber and nutrients. Enjoy these spiced pears, which are poached to tasty perfection.

2 cups white wine, preferably dry	1 (2-inch) piece of ginger, sliced	Juice and grated zest of 2 oranges	4 Bosc pears, peeled, cored, and quartered
1 cinnamon stick	5 cardamom pods		

1. Cut a piece of parchment paper into a circle slightly smaller in size than the saucepan you are using and punch a small hole in its center.
2. In the medium saucepan, stir together the white wine, cinnamon, ginger, cardamom, and orange juice and zest on high heat. Bring to just before a boil, lower the heat so the liquid simmers, and add the pears.
3. Place the parchment paper over the pears. (This will keep just enough pressure for the pears to stay beneath the level of the poaching liquid and still allow steam to escape.)
4. Poach the pears for at least 20 minutes. The more time you have, the more flavor they will absorb.
5. Remove the pears from poaching liquid with a slotted spoon. Eat as is or return the poaching liquid (without the pears) to a simmer until the liquid reduces to a syrupy sauce, about 10 minutes. Strain the sauce and pour it over the poached pears.

Storage Tip:

Store the pears in an airtight container in the refrigerator for up to 4 days.

Variation:

The Bosc pear is great for both its flavor and its ability to hold its shape during the poaching process, although the Anjou, Concorde, and French butter pears are also quite lovely. Avoid Comice and Bartlett pears if you can when making this recipe, because they don't hold up as well.

Per Serving: Calories: 228; Total fat: <1g; Saturated fat: 0g; Sodium: 8g; Total carbohydrates: 35g; Sugar: 22g; Fiber: 6g; Net carbohydrates: 29g; Protein: 1g

Raspberry Coconut Bliss Balls

30 MINUTES OR LESS, GLUTEN-FREE, SOY-FREE, VEGAN

Makes 12 balls

Prep time: 10 minutes, plus 15 minutes soaking time

Sweetened naturally with dates, these delightful bites are loaded with healthy fats, natural sweetness, fiber, and oh so much delicious flavor. Coconut and raspberry are an unlikely pair, but they create a harmonious blend, especially if you are a fan of super simple bite-size treats.

¼ cup pitted dates (about 2 ounces)

½ cup almond flour

¾ cup unsweetened shredded coconut, divided

½ cup frozen raspberries

1. In a small bowl, cover the dates with hot water. Let them sit for 15 minutes to soften. Drain.
2. In a food processor, combine the almond flour, ½ cup shredded coconut, and the raspberries and dates. Process until they're smooth.
3. Remove the dough and roll it into 12 (1-inch) balls. Place the remaining ¼ cup of coconut in a small bowl and roll the balls in it to coat.

Storage Tip:

Refrigerate in an airtight container for up to 4 days.

Per Serving (2 balls): Calories: 114; Total fat: 7g; Saturated fat: 3g; Sodium: 4mg; Total carbohydrates: 11g; Sugar: 7g; Fiber: 3g; Net carbohydrates: 8g; Protein: 3g

Raw Chocolate Truffles

30 MINUTES OR LESS, GLUTEN-FREE, SOY-FREE, VEGAN

Makes 12 truffles   **Prep time:** 15 minutes

These gooey, chewy, deliciously rich truffles are made with naturally occurring sugar found in raisins. Raisins are a good source of fiber, which is crucial for promoting healthy blood sugar levels. If you are allergic to cashews, substitute your favorite raw seeds or nuts. For an extra-chocolaty flavor, add an extra 1 to 2 tablespoons of cocoa or cacao powder.

2 cups raisins

2 tablespoons water

1 cup raw cashews

1 tablespoon cocoa powder

1 teaspoon ground cinnamon

½ teaspoon vanilla extract

½ cup pumpkin seeds

¼ teaspoon kosher salt

1. Combine the raisins and water in a food processor and pulse until a paste is formed.
2. Add the cashews, cocoa powder, cinnamon, and vanilla to the food processor and pulse until a paste is formed.
3. Add the pumpkin seeds and salt to the mixture and pulse until the pumpkin seeds are chopped. (Do not overprocess. You don't want the pumpkin seeds to turn into a paste.)
4. Use a spoon to scoop about 2 teaspoons of mixture and form 12 small balls using your hands. Place on parchment paper, spaced 1 inch apart.
5. Store in an airtight container in the refrigerator or at room temperature.

Variation:

You can add different spices to change up the flavor. A quarter teaspoon of powdered ginger, cardamom, and nutmeg all work great! Optionally, you can roll the truffle balls in ½ cup of cocoa powder, powdered sugar, or sesame seeds for added taste.

Per Serving (1 truffle): Calories: 172; Total fat: 8g; Saturated fat: 1g; Sodium: 538mg; Total carbohydrates: 24g; Sugar: 15g; Fiber: 11g; Net carbohydrates: 13g; Protein: 10g

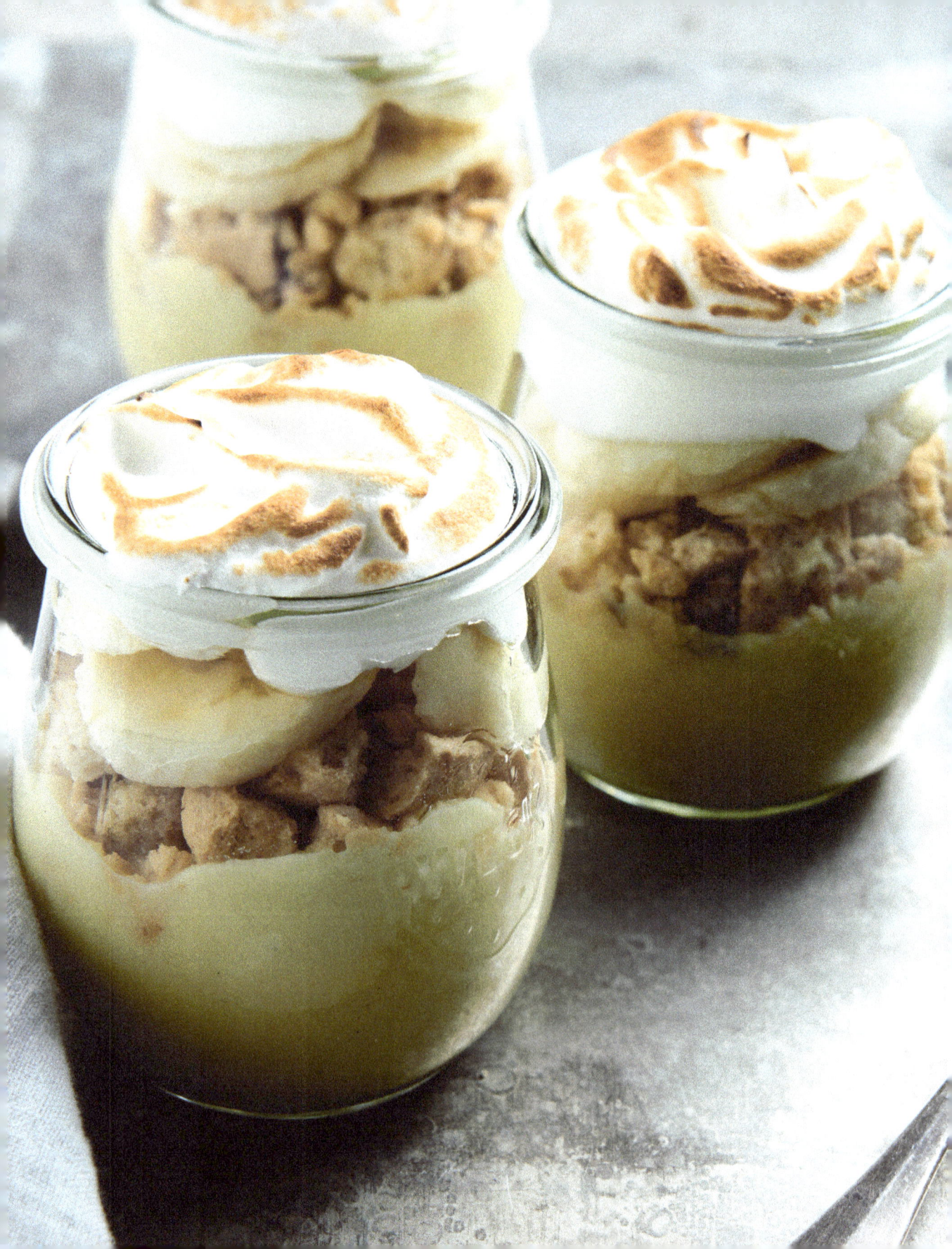

Banana Pudding

SOY-FREE, VEGETARIAN

Serves 8
Prep time: 30 minutes

Cook time: 20 minutes

In this diabetes-friendly banana pudding, the sugar, carbohydrates, and saturated fat are reduced while keeping the creamy and luxurious texture and taste. Vanilla wafers pair nicely with the banana in this recipe, but if you'd like to reduce the carbs, you can swap for any low-carb cookie instead. If you'd like, you can make these as individual servings and toast the meringue topping with a kitchen torch instead of putting it in the oven.

1 cup erythritol or stevia

5 teaspoons almond flour

¼ teaspoon kosher salt

2½ cups fat-free milk

6 tablespoons prepared egg replacement

1 teaspoon vanilla extract

10 vanilla wafers, crushed

5 medium bananas, sliced

5 medium egg whites (1 cup)

1. In a saucepan, whisk ¾ cup of the erythritol, almond flour, salt, and milk together. Cook over medium heat until the sugar is dissolved.
2. Whisk in the egg replacement and cook for about 10 minutes, or until thickened.
3. Remove from the heat and stir in the ½ teaspoon of the vanilla.
4. Spread the thickened pudding onto the bottom of a 10-inch square casserole dish.
5. Spread the crushed wafers on top of the pudding.
6. Place a layer of sliced bananas on top of the wafers.
7. Preheat the oven to 350°F.
8. In a medium bowl, beat the egg whites for about 5 minutes, or until stiff.
9. Add the remaining ¼ cup of erythritol and the remaining ½ teaspoon of vanilla while continuing to beat for about 3 more minutes.
10. Spread the meringue on top of the banana pudding.
11. Transfer the casserole dish to the oven, and bake for 7 to 10 minutes, or until the top is lightly browned.

Per Serving: Calories: 138; Total fat: 2g; Saturated fat: 0g; Sodium: 141mg; Total carbohydrates: 24g; Sugar: 14g; Fiber: 2g; Net carbohydrates: 22g; Protein: 7g

Chocolate Tahini Bombs

30 MINUTES OR LESS, GLUTEN-FREE, VEGETARIAN

Makes 15 bombs
Prep time: 20 minutes

Cook time: 8 minutes

Sesame is the unsung hero of the dessert world and a healthier way to enjoy something sweet. Tahini, the ground product of toasted sesame seeds, contains more protein than milk and most nuts. This fragrant paste is a rich source of B vitamins, which boost energy and brain function; vitamin E, which helps fight heart disease and stroke; and minerals like magnesium, iron, and calcium. It's amazing to find all this nutritional power in a simple dessert.

15 whole dates, pits removed (date intact, not split in half completely)

2½ tablespoons tahini, divided

½ cup canned full-fat coconut milk

4 ounces dark chocolate, chopped

1 tablespoon toasted sesame seeds

1. Line a baking sheet with parchment paper.
2. Fill each date with a small amount of the tahini, roughly ¼ teaspoon, and place them on the prepared baking sheet. Put the filled dates in the freezer for 10 to 15 minutes.
3. Meanwhile, in a small saucepan over medium-low heat, heat the coconut milk until simmering.
4. Place the chocolate in a medium heatproof bowl, and when the milk is simmering, pour it into the bowl and let stand for 3 minutes to soften the chocolate.
5. Stir the mixture until it is smooth and the chocolate is completely melted.
6. Remove the dates from the freezer and dip one date at a time into the chocolate. Coat evenly using a fork and place them back on the baking sheet. Sprinkle the dates with the sesame seeds and repeat until all dates are coated in chocolate.
7. Allow to cool completely for the chocolate to harden or eat immediately.

Prep Tip:

If the chocolate is not melting, do not put it in the microwave! Place the bowl in a saucepan filled with a few inches of gently simmering water over low heat and stir the chocolate until it melts.

Per Serving (1 bomb): Calories: 97; Total fat: 6g; Saturated fat: 3g; Sodium: 9mg; Carbohydrates: 10g; Sugar: 6g; Fiber: 2g; Net carbohydrates: 8g; Protein: 1g

Ambrosia

GLUTEN-FREE, SOY-FREE, VEGETARIAN

Serves 8   **Prep time:** 10 minutes, plus overnight to set

Often present on the Southern holiday table, ambrosia is a sweet dish that's simple to make and has been aptly called "the fruit of the gods." Mixing tropical fruits with standard oranges, this recipe substitutes the expected pineapple with peaches, a fruit that's local to the South, but keeps the coconut for a textured, refreshing bite.

3 oranges, peeled, sectioned, and quartered

2 (4-ounce) cups diced peaches in water, drained

1 cup shredded, unsweetened coconut

1 (8-ounce) container fat-free crème fraîche

In a large mixing bowl, combine the oranges, peaches, coconut, and crème fraîche. Gently toss until well mixed. Cover and refrigerate overnight.

Prep Tip:

If you can't find peaches in water, buy peaches packed in 100% juice, and rinse them well before using.

Per Serving (¼ cup): Calories: 97; Total fat: 4g; Saturated fat: 1g; Sodium: 7mg; Total carbohydrates: 16g; Sugar: 8g; Fiber: 3g; Net carbohydrates: 13g; Protein: 2g

Fried Apples

30 MINUTES OR LESS, GLUTEN-FREE, NUT-FREE, SOY-FREE, VEGAN

Serves 4
Prep time: 5 minutes

Cook time: 10 minutes

Fried apples are a perfect Southern tradition. And this recipe is a healthy spin that doesn't use butter. This classic comfort food that you can make in 15 minutes is delicious by itself or when used as a pie filling.

4 medium Pink Lady apples (or any apples you like), quartered

Avocado oil, for brushing

¼ cup erythritol or other brown sugar replacement

1. Brush the apple pieces with avocado oil. In a small mixing bowl, toss them in the erythritol.
2. In a large skillet over medium heat, panfry the apple pieces, turning occasionally, until they are caramelized on all sides, about 10 minutes.

Prep Tip:

When choosing a sugar replacement, it's important to look for a natural sweetener that bakes similarly to table sugar and won't produce unwanted gastrointestinal side effects.

Per Serving (1 apple): Calories: 97; Total fat: 3g; Saturated fat: 0g; Sodium: 1mg; Total carbohydrates: 28g; Sugar: 14g; Fiber: 3g; Net carbohydrates: 25g; Protein: 0g;

Cheesecake-Stuffed Strawberries

30 MINUTES OR LESS, NUT-FREE, SOY-FREE, VEGETARIAN

Serves 4   **Prep time:** 15 minutes

This is a lovely dessert to serve to guests, as these stuffed strawberries look rather elegant on a platter. For added flair, use a piping bag or simply put the filling in a resealable plastic bag, cut a small piece from a bottom corner, and pipe the filling into the strawberries. To lower the carbs even more, use 1 tablespoon of a granulated sweetener of choice in place of the maple syrup—and the graham cracker crumbles are optional.

12 large strawberries

4 ounces low-fat cream cheese, at room temperature

1 tablespoon pure maple syrup or honey

1 teaspoon vanilla extract

2 tablespoons graham cracker crumbs (optional)

1. Using a paring knife, cut the tops off the strawberries and hollow them out to make a hole for the filling. Set aside.
2. In a medium bowl, using a handheld electric mixer on medium, beat the cream cheese, maple syrup, and vanilla until smooth. Spoon or pipe the filling into the strawberries and arrange on a tray.
3. Sprinkle with graham cracker crumbs (if using).

Storage Tip:

Refrigerate in an airtight container for up to 3 days.

Per Serving (3 strawberries): Calories: 90; Total fat: 5g; Saturated fat: 3g; Sodium: 103mg; Total carbohydrates: 10g; Sugar: 7g; Fiber: 1g; Net carbohydrates: 9g; Protein: 3g

Lime, Mint, Orange Yogurt Parfait

30 MINUTES OR LESS, GLUTEN-FREE, NUT-FREE, SOY-FREE, VEGETARIAN

Serves 4 | **Prep time:** 10 minutes

Parfaits are easy desserts that can be completely customized to anyone's taste. This simple version uses a mix of orange, lime, and mint, but you can use any combination of fruit and citrus juice. Grapefruit, blackberries, blueberries, and strawberries are all delightful substitutes for the mandarin oranges.

2 cups plain low-fat Greek yogurt

Juice and grated zest of 1 lime

2 tablespoons granulated sweetener of choice

1 (8-ounce) can mandarin oranges in juice, drained

4 or 5 fresh mint leaves, chopped

1. In a large bowl, mix the yogurt, lime juice and zest, and sweetener.
2. Into four small glasses, add a few segments of oranges. Divide the yogurt between the glasses and top with the remaining orange slices. Sprinkle the mint leaves over the top of the parfaits.

Storage Tip:

Refrigerate the parfaits, covered, for up to 3 days.

Per Serving: Calories: 96; Total fat: 2g; Saturated fat: 1g; Sodium: 88mg; Total carbohydrates: 13g; Sugar: 12g; Fiber: 1g; Net carbohydrates: 12g; Protein: 7g

Peach and Almond Meal Fritters

30 MINUTES OR LESS, DAIRY-FREE, GLUTEN-FREE, SOY-FREE, VEGETARIAN

Serves 7
Prep time: 15 minutes

Cook time: 15 minutes

These fritters are the perfect balance of savory and sweet. The almond meal and eggs offer a good balance of heart-healthy fats and protein paired with the sweet, nutrient-rich fruits. Although this is a dessert, you could alternatively serve it at breakfast with eggs and greens of your choice.

4 ripe bananas, mashed

2 cups chopped peaches

1 medium egg

2 medium egg whites

¾ cup almond meal

¼ teaspoon almond extract

1 tablespoon avocado oil

1. In a large bowl, mash the bananas and peaches together with a fork or potato masher.
2. Blend in the whole egg and egg whites. Stir in the almond meal and almond extract.
3. In a large skillet on medium heat, heat the sunflower oil. Working in batches, drop ¼-cup portions of the batter into the skillet and cook until the edges become brown. Turn the fritters and cook the other side until browned, about 8 minutes in total
4. Repeat with the remaining batter and serve.

Per Serving (2 fritters): Calories: 168; Total fat: 8g; Saturated fat: 1g; Sodium: 23mg; Total carbohydrates: 22g; Sugar: 12g; Fiber: 4g; Net carbohydrates: 18g; Protein: 6g

Chocolate Pudding

GLUTEN-FREE, VEGAN

Serves 4

Prep time: 5 minutes, plus 30 minutes to chill

Cook time: 2 minutes

Chocolate pudding is always a welcomed treat! This alternative using silken tofu is a delight, as everyone will ooh and ahh over its smooth, rich taste. Company will think you worked for hours perfecting it, but you'll know all it took was mere minutes.

4 ounces chopped semisweet chocolate

1 (12-ounce) block silken tofu, drained, at room temperature

Whipped coconut cream, for topping (optional)

Berries, for topping (optional)

Mini chocolate chips, for topping (optional; vegan if necessary)

1. Place the chocolate in a microwave-safe bowl and melt in the microwave in 30 second intervals, stirring after each. Set the chocolate aside to cool.
2. Place the silken tofu in a blender and blend until smooth. Add the melted chocolate and blend until smooth and creamy.
3. Transfer the pudding to 4 serving bowls, cover, and refrigerate for 30 minutes or up to 3 days. Serve topped with desired garnishes.

Per Serving: Calories: 216; Total fat: 14g; Saturated fat: 0g; Sodium: 30mg; Carbohydrates: 16g; Sugar: 11g; Fiber: 4g; Net carbohydrates: 12g; Protein: 7g

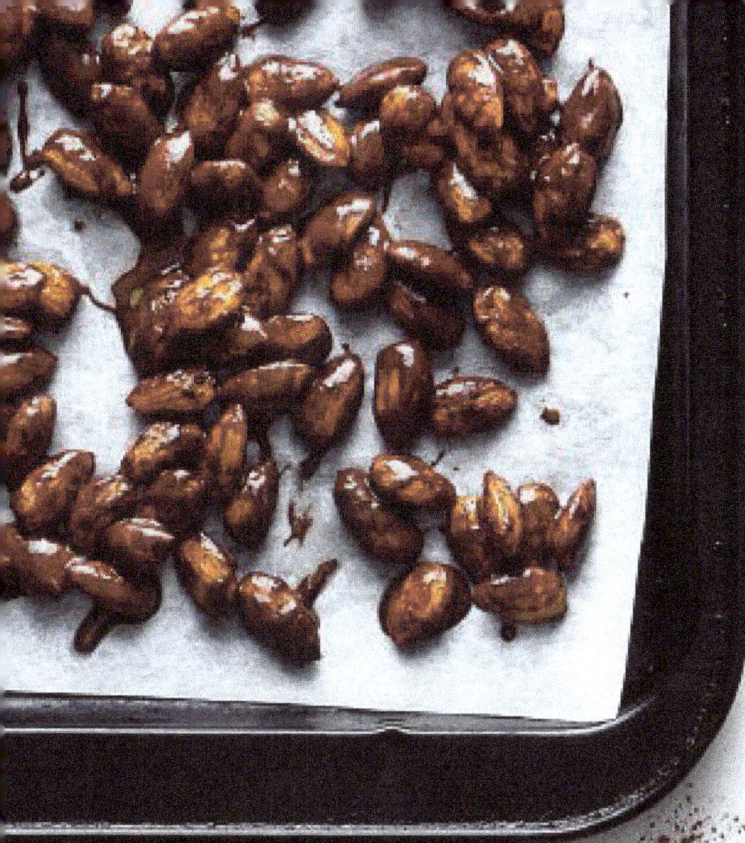

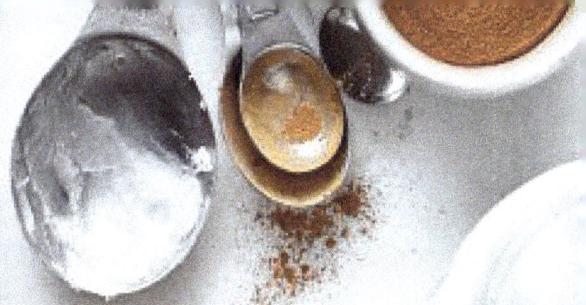

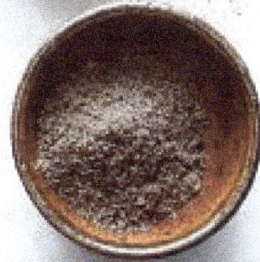

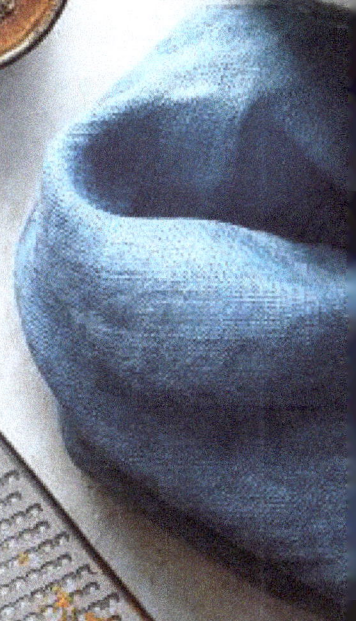

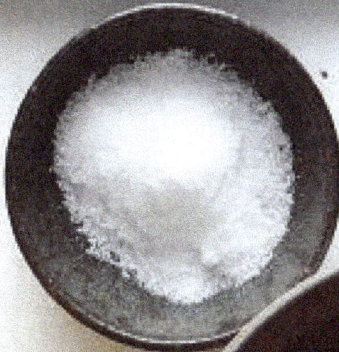

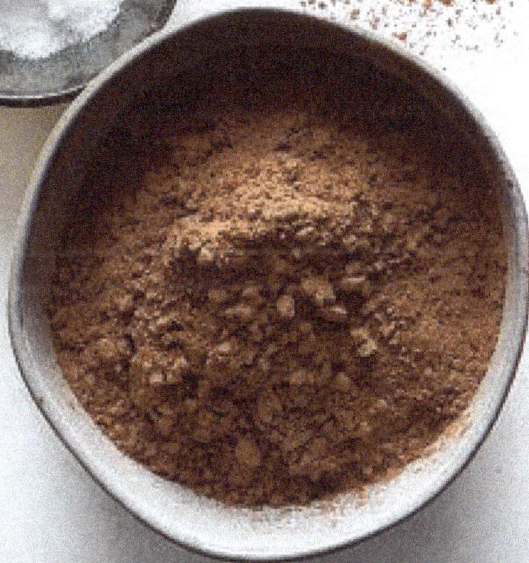

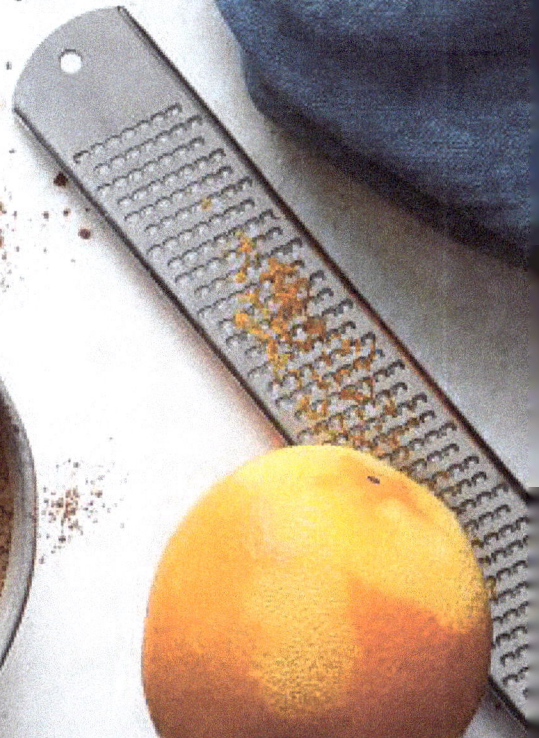

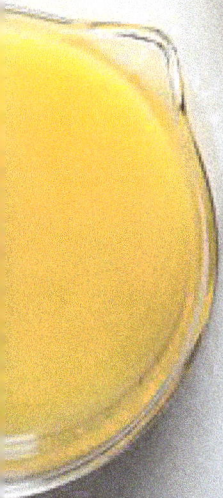

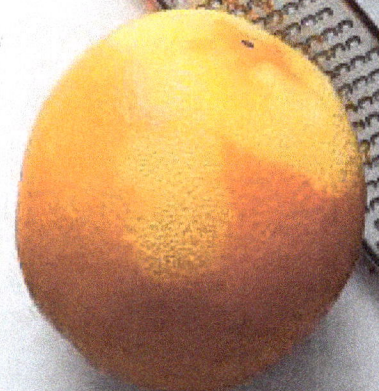

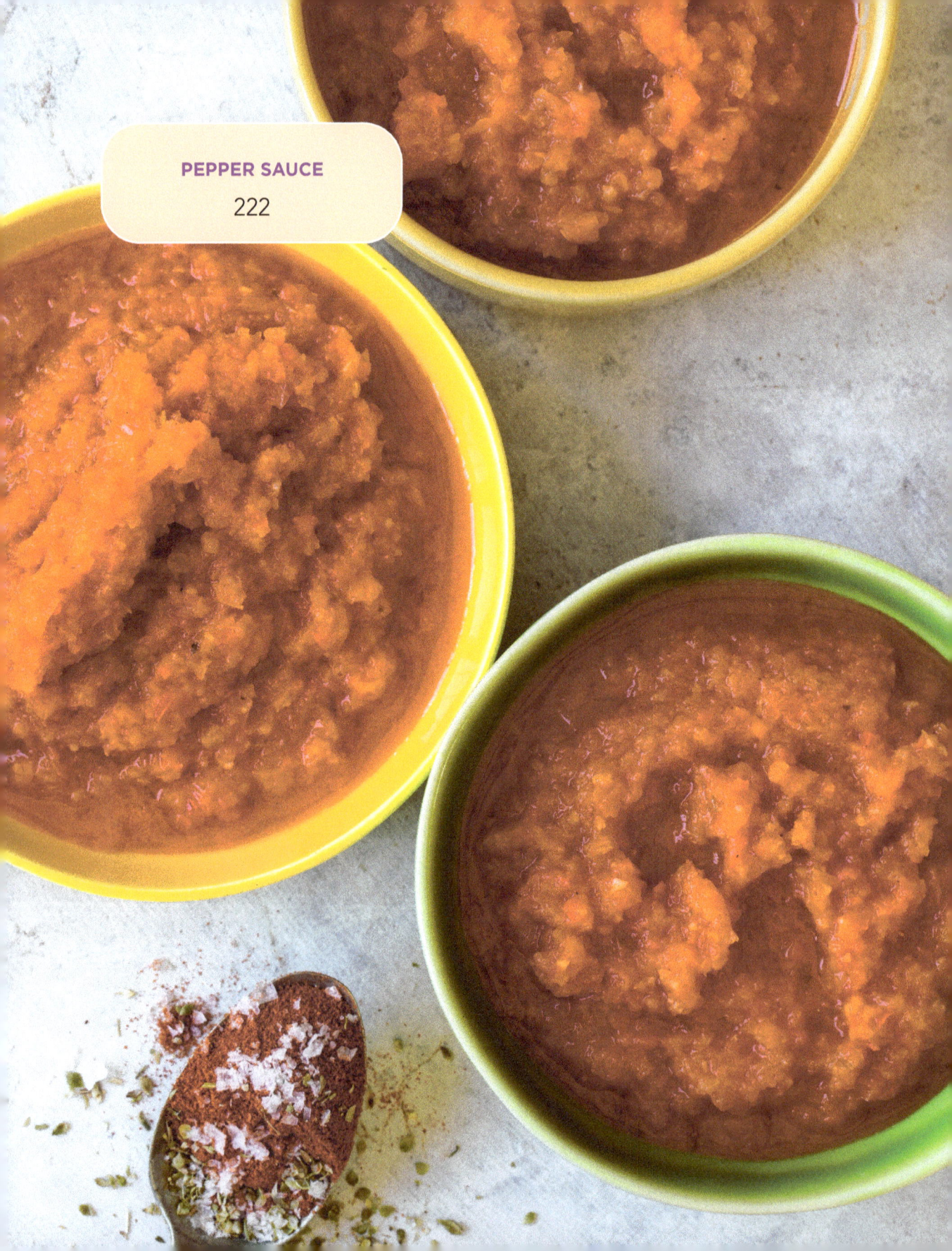

PEPPER SAUCE

222

9

SAUCES AND STAPLES

Quick Pickled Vegetables

GLUTEN-FREE, NUT-FREE, SOY-FREE, VEGAN

Makes 4 (12- to 16-ounce) jars pickles

Prep time: 10 minutes, plus 24 hours in the refrigerator

Pickles add a distinctive crunch and tang to any dish, and they range from sweet to spicy depending on the flavorful brine you choose. You can use and customize this quick pickle brine to pickle almost any vegetable you love.

1 tablespoon whole allspice

1 teaspoon black peppercorns

1 tablespoon whole mustard seeds

1 teaspoon celery seeds

4 garlic cloves, smashed

7 to 10 whole okra

1 sweet onion, quartered

1 cup green beans

3 Kirby cucumbers, cut into ½-inch-thick rounds

4 cups vinegar

4 cups boiling water

1. In a small bowl, to make the dry mixture, combine the allspice, peppercorns, mustard seeds, and celery seeds.
2. Into each of four (12- to 16-ounce) heatproof jars, add 1 teaspoon of the dry mixture.
3. Add 1 garlic clove to each jar.
4. Fill one jar with okra, one with onion, one with green beans, and the last with cucumbers.
5. In a large bowl, mix the vinegar and boiling water.
6. Fill each jar with the vinegar and water mixture up to three-quarters full. Cover and let stand for 30 minutes, or until room temperature, then refrigerate for at least 24 hours.

Storage Tip:

Refrigerate the pickles for up to 2 months.

Prep Tip:

Double the quantity to make extra!

Per Serving: Calories: 137; Total fat: 1g; Saturated fat: 0g; Sodium: 25mg; Total carbohydrates: 21g; Sugar: 7g; Fiber: 4g; Net carbohydrates: 17g; Protein: 4g

Cauliflower Rice

GLUTEN-FREE, NUT-FREE, SOY-FREE, VEGAN, 30 MINUTES OR LESS

Makes 2½ cups
Prep time: 5 minutes

Cook time: 5 minutes

Cauliflower rice cooks much faster than regular rice, so it can cut down on the cooking time if you use it in dishes like the Cauli-Lettuce Wraps (page 89). This side dish is also a wonderful replacement for grains in general, especially when you have other carbohydrates in your meal that could cross over into excessive amounts.

1½ pounds cauliflower, coarsely chopped

½ tablespoon extra-virgin olive oil

Kosher salt

Freshly ground black pepper

1. Pulse the cauliflower in a food processor until it has a crumbly texture, almost like rice. Be careful not to over-pulse and make it too fine. It's okay to have some larger chunks. Another option is to use a box grater if you don't have a food processor. Put the crumbled cauliflower in a bowl and set aside.
2. In a large skillet over medium-high heat, heat the olive oil. Add the cauliflower, stir to coat with the oil, and sauté 3 to 5 minutes. Season with salt and pepper and serve.

Storage Tip:

Refrigerate any leftovers in an airtight container for 3 to 4 days.

Variation:

Add any spice blend you want to jazz up the flavor of the cauliflower rice. Try curry powder or add some fresh cilantro with lime, or fresh parsley with lemon.

Per Serving (½ cup): Calories: 46; Total fat: 2g; Saturated fat: 0g; Sodium: 72mg; Total carbohydrates: 7g; Sugar: 3g; Fiber: 3g; Net carbohydrates: 4g; Protein: 3g

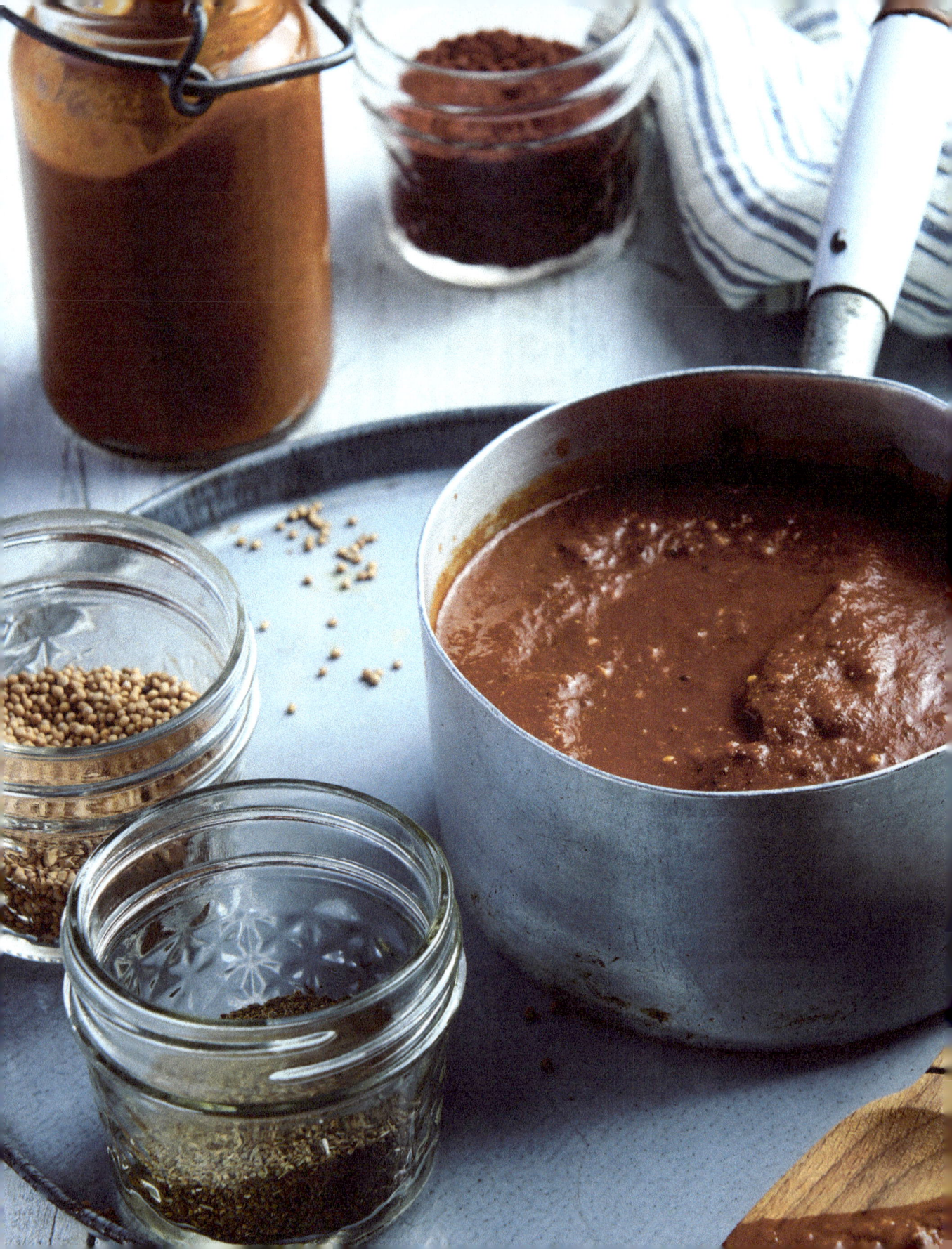

Barbecue Sauce

30 MINUTES OR LESS, GLUTEN-FREE, NUT-FREE, SOY-FREE, VEGAN

Makes ~3 cups
Prep time: 5 minutes

Cook time: 15 minutes

The culinary roots of barbecue come from the Caribbean, where the tradition of slow-cooking meat over a low and indirect heat source was born. Spanish conquistadors named the indigenous style of cooking barbacoa and brought the technique with them as they occupied northern territories. Over time, barbecue has transformed and varies regionally.

1½ cups white vinegar

1¼ cups tomato puree

1 tablespoon yellow mustard

1 teaspoon mustard seeds

1 teaspoon ground turmeric

1 teaspoon sweet paprika

1 teaspoon garlic powder

1 teaspoon celery seeds

½ teaspoon cayenne pepper

½ teaspoon onion powder

½ teaspoon freshly ground black pepper

1. In a medium pot, combine the vinegar, tomato puree, mustard, mustard seeds, turmeric, paprika, garlic powder, celery seeds, cayenne, onion powder, and black pepper. Simmer over low heat for 15 minutes, or until the flavors come together.
2. Remove the sauce from the heat and let cool for 5 minutes. Transfer to a blender, and puree until smooth.

Storage Tip:

Freeze leftover barbecue sauce in an ice cube tray and place in a sealed freezer-proof container.

Per Serving (2 tablespoons): Calories: 7; Total fat: 0g; Saturated fat: 0g; Sodium: 12mg; Total carbohydrates: 2g; Sugar: 1g; Fiber: 0g; Net carbohydrates: 2g; Protein: 0g

Peanut Sauce

30 MINUTES OR LESS, DAIRY-FREE, GLUTEN-FREE, ONE-POT, VEGETARIAN

Makes 1 to 1¼ cups   **Prep time:** 5 to 10 minutes

Peanut butter, and peanuts, in general, have gotten a lot of love over the years. Peanut sauce is used in pan-Asian dishes, especially those developed by Thai and Laotian immigrants and other members of the Southeast Asian diaspora. This peanut sauce is a nod to this tradition and works well on everything, such as noodles, chicken, salad, and rice.

½ cup unsalted, unsweetened creamy peanut butter

2 tablespoons reduced-sodium soy sauce or tamari

1 tablespoon honey

2 garlic cloves, minced

1 teaspoon diced chile

Juice of 1 lime

In a medium bowl, whisk together the peanut butter, soy sauce, honey, garlic, chile, and lime juice until thoroughly combined. Add water to thin out the consistency. Taste and adjust the seasonings as desired.

Storage Tip:

Refrigerate in an airtight container for up to 1 week or freeze for up to 3 months.

Per Serving (2 tablespoons): Calories: 87; Total fat: 7g; Saturated fat: 1g; Sodium: 105mg; Total carbohydrates: 5g; Sugar: 3g; Fiber: 1g; Net carbohydrates: 4g; Protein: 3g

Pea Pesto

30 MINUTES OR LESS, GLUTEN-FREE, ONE-POT, SOY-FREE, VEGETARIAN

Serves 4   **Prep time:** 5 minutes

It's important to use fresh green peas here, which have the right flavor and texture to make this work. Frozen peas have too high of a water content and will result in a watery pesto. You can also use edamame if you wish.

½ cup fresh green peas

½ cup grated Parmesan cheese

¼ cup fresh basil leaves

¼ cup extra-virgin olive oil

¼ cup pine nuts

2 garlic cloves, minced

¼ teaspoon kosher salt

In a blender or food processor, combine all the ingredients. Process until smooth.

Storage Tip:

The sauce will store well in the refrigerator for up to 2 days. You can also freeze it in ice cube trays for use in other dishes and sauces. The frozen cubes will last in the freezer for 6 months.

Variation:

You can try this with edamame without changing the carbohydrate count significantly.

Per Serving: Calories: 248; Total fat: 23g; Saturated fat: 3g; Sodium: 338mg; Total carbohydrates: 5g; Sugar: 1g; Fiber: 1g; Net carbohydrates: 4g; Protein: 7g

Italian/Greek Vinaigrette

30 MINUTES OR LESS, GLUTEN-FREE, NUT-FREE, VEGAN

Serves 4   **Prep time:** 5 minutes

This basic recipe allows you to make two different vinaigrettes: Italian and Greek. Carb counts are about the same for each, as is the process for making them. The only difference is in the ingredients.

For Italian dressing

¼ cup extra-virgin olive oil

2 tablespoons red wine vinegar

1 tablespoon minced shallot

2 teaspoons Italian seasoning

1 garlic clove, finely minced

1 teaspoon Dijon mustard

¼ teaspoon kosher salt

⅛ teaspoon freshly ground black pepper

For Greek dressing

¼ cup extra virgin olive oil

1 tablespoon red wine vinegar

1 tablespoon freshly squeezed lemon juice

3 garlic cloves, minced

1 teaspoon dried oregano

1 teaspoon dried marjoram

½ teaspoon grated lemon zest

¼ teaspoon kosher salt

For both dressings, in a small bowl, whisk all the ingredients together until well combined.

Storage Tip:

Refrigerate the vinaigrettes for up to 5 days. Whisk before using.

Variation:

Add heat to either dressing with a pinch of red pepper flakes.

Per Serving: Calories: 127; Total fat: 14g; Saturated fat: 2g; Sodium: 74mg; Total carbohydrates: 1g; Sugar: 0g; Fiber: <1g; Net carbohydrates: 1g; Protein: 0g

Creamy Ranch Dressing

30 MINUTES OR LESS, GLUTEN-FREE, NUT-FREE, ONE-POT, VEGETARIAN

Serves 4   **Prep time:** 10 minutes

Who doesn't like a good, creamy ranch dressing? But store-bought versions can be quite processed and full of fat. To keep the creamy richness without the excess calories, make your own—with less fat yet tons of flavor thanks to the variety of herbs. For those of you who prefer a thicker dressing, add half the milk first, then adjust as desired.

¾ cup fat-free sour cream

½ cup plain nonfat Greek yogurt

Juice of ½ lemon

2 teaspoons dried chives

2 teaspoons dried parsley

1 teaspoon kosher salt

1 teaspoon garlic powder

1 teaspoon onion powder

1 cup skim milk

Freshly ground black pepper

1. In a small bowl, stir together the sour cream and yogurt.
2. Add the lemon juice, chives, parsley, salt, garlic powder, and onion powder, and stir well to combine.
3. Whisk in the milk until smooth, and season with pepper. Transfer to a jar, cover, and refrigerate for up to 2 weeks.

Per Serving: Calories: 78; Total fat: 0g; Saturated fat: 0g; Sodium: 379mg; Total carbohydrates: 13g; Sugar: 4g; Fiber: 0g; Net carbohydrates: 13g; Protein: 7g

Balsamic Vinaigrette

30 MINUTES OR LESS, GLUTEN-FREE, NUT-FREE, ONE-POT, VEGAN

Makes ~1 cup   Prep time: 5 minutes

Ditch the store-bought dressings for this easy vinaigrette, which may be the best you've ever had. The nice thing about vinaigrettes is how versatile they are. Swap out balsamic for red wine vinegar or even freshly squeezed lemon juice. No matter how you like it, this vinaigrette will become a staple in your fridge.

¾ cup extra-virgin olive oil

¼ cup balsamic vinegar
2 garlic cloves, minced

1 teaspoon Dijon mustard

½ teaspoon freshly ground black pepper
¼ teaspoon kosher salt

In a small bowl or lidded jar, combine the olive oil, vinegar, garlic, mustard, pepper, and salt. Whisk to combine or cover and shake until blended. Keep covered and refrigerate for up to 1 month.

Per Serving (2 tablespoons): Calories: 171; Total fat: 19g; Saturated fat: 3g; Sodium: 83mg; Carbohydrates: 2g; Sugar: 1g; Fiber: 0g; Net carbohydrates: 2g; Protein: 0g;

Tomato, Caper, and Golden Raisin Sauce

30 MINUTES OR LESS, GLUTEN-FREE, NUT-FREE, ONE-POT, SOY-FREE, VEGAN

Makes ~4 cups
Prep time: 5 minutes

Cook time: 25 minutes

Although this Mediterranean-based sauce is used in the Cauliflower Steaks recipe (page 133), it also pairs beautifully with meats like beef, lamb, or chicken and even fish like swordfish and halibut. One could also use it in place of marinara sauce when making pasta for a little more sweetness and an enticing, distinct dish.

2 tablespoons extra-virgin olive oil	1 (28-ounce) can crushed tomatoes	1 teaspoon dried oregano	Pinch freshly ground black pepper
6 garlic cloves, minced	¼ cup golden raisins	Pinch kosher salt	3 fresh basil leaves
	2 tablespoons capers		

1. In a large saucepan over medium heat, heat the olive oil. Sauté the garlic until softened, about 3 minutes. Add the tomatoes, raisins, capers, oregano, salt, and pepper and bring the sauce to a simmer. Add the basil leaves, including the stem, and allow them to wilt, then submerge the leaves in the sauce.
2. Simmer the sauce until thickened, about 15 minutes.

Storage Tip:

Refrigerate in an airtight container for up to 1 week or freeze for up to 3 months.

Variation:

Make the sauce even more exciting with the addition of salty anchovies, olives, or dried herbs such as marjoram, tarragon, parsley, and thyme.

Per Serving (½ cup): Calories: 82; Total fat: 4g; Saturated fat: 1g; Sodium: 185mg; Total carbohydrates: 12g; Sugar: 6g; Fiber: 2g; Net carbohydrates: 10g; Protein: 2g

Pepper Sauce

30 MINUTES OR LESS, NUT-FREE, SOY-FREE, VEGAN

Makes 4 cups
Prep time: 10 minutes

Cook time: 20 minutes

This pepper sauce is a spin on the sauces found throughout the Caribbean. Make the sauce fiery by leaving the seeds in the peppers when cooking or seed them to reduce the heat. The spice will be dependent on the chiles, so if you're looking for a milder hot sauce, use a deseeded jalapeño pepper or serrano pepper. If you really love the burn, go for a Scotch bonnet or ghost pepper.

2 red hot fresh
  chiles, seeded
2 dried chiles

½ small yellow onion,
  coarsely chopped
2 garlic cloves, peeled

2 cups water
2 cups white vinegar

1. In a medium saucepan, combine the fresh and dried chiles, onion, garlic, and water. Bring to a simmer and cook for 20 minutes, or until tender. Transfer to a food processor or blender.
2. Add the vinegar and blend until smooth.

Storage Tip:

Refrigerate in an airtight container for up to 3 months.

Per Serving (2 tablespoons): Calories: 2; Total fat: 0g; Saturated fat: 0g; Sodium: 1mg; Total carbohydrates: 0g; Sugar: 0g; Fiber: 0g; Net carbohydrates: 0g; Protein: 0g

Peri-Peri Sauce (Piri-Piri)

30 MINUTES OR LESS, GLUTEN-FREE, NUT-FREE, SOY-FREE, VEGAN

Serves 4
Prep time: 10 minutes

Cook time: 5 minutes

This South African sauce adds tremendous zip to all kinds of foods, including fish and seafood, poultry, meat, and tofu. This is a relatively low-heat version, so feel free to add additional spicy chiles to adjust to your own personal heat preferences.

1 red bell pepper, seeded and chopped

1 red onion, chopped

1 tomato, chopped

4 garlic cloves, minced

1 red chile, seeded and chopped

2 tablespoons extra-virgin olive oil

Juice of 1 lemon

1 tablespoon smoked paprika

1 tablespoon dried oregano

1 teaspoon kosher salt

1. In a blender or food processor, combine all the ingredients. Process until smooth.
2. In a small saucepan over medium-high heat, bring the mixture to a simmer, stirring constantly. Reduce the heat to medium and simmer for 5 minutes.

Storage Tip:

The sauce will store well in the refrigerator for up to 5 days. You can also freeze it in ice cube trays in tablespoon sizes for use in other dishes and sauces. The frozen cubes will last in the freezer for 6 months.

Variation:

Along with adjusting this recipe by using more or spicier chiles, you can also adjust the heat levels upward by adding cayenne or downward by omitting the fresh chile.

Per Serving: Calories: 99; Total fat: 7g; Saturated fat: 1g; Sodium: 296mg; Total carbohydrates: 8g; Sugar: 2g; Fiber: 3g; Net carbohydrates: 5g; Protein: 1g

Pub Sauce

30 MINUTES OR LESS, DAIRY-FREE, NUT-FREE, VEGETARIAN

Serves 4   **Prep time:** 5 minutes

This pub sauce is delicious on just about any burger. It also makes a great base for tuna or crab salad, a tasty dip for veggies, or a yummy side dip for chicken fingers or fish sticks.

¼ cup mayonnaise

1 tablespoon pure maple syrup

1 tablespoon reduced-sodium soy sauce

1 tablespoon Worcestershire sauce

1 garlic clove, minced

In a small bowl, whisk all the ingredients until well combined.

Storage Tip:

Refrigerate the sauce for up to 3 days.

Variation:

Add chopped fresh herbs, such as chives, if you wish to pump up the flavor. Adding up to 1 tablespoon of chopped fresh herbs changes the flavor but will not have a significant effect on carbohydrate counts or how you dose insulin.

Per Serving: Calories: 113; Total fat: 10g; Saturated fat: 2g; Sodium: 257mg; Total carbohydrates: 5g; Sugar: 4g; Fiber: 0g; Net carbohydrates: 5g; Protein: 1g

Broth Three Ways (Vegetable, Chicken, and Seafood)

DAIRY-FREE, GLUTEN-FREE, NUT-FREE, SOY-FREE

Serves 8
Prep time: 10 minutes

Cook time: 35 minutes

Homemade broth may sound intimidating, but these variations, all made in a pressure cooker, remove the guesswork. You can also make any of these by simmering them on low in a covered pot for one to two hours.

For the vegetable broth

1 whole garlic bulb	3 large carrots, halved	2 fresh rosemary sprigs	8 cups water
1 large unpeeled yellow onion, halved	1 bunch collard greens, coarsely chopped	2 fresh parsley sprigs	
3 celery stalks, halved	2 bay leaves	1 (1-inch) piece fresh ginger	

For the chicken broth

1 whole chicken carcass	1 large unpeeled yellow onion, halved	3 large carrots, halved	2 bay leaves
1 whole garlic bulb	3 celery stalks, halved	1 large beefsteak tomato, quartered	2 fresh thyme sprigs
			8 cups water

For the seafood broth

1 quart shrimp shells (or 1 whole fish with bones)	1 large unpeeled yellow onion, halved	2 fresh parsley sprigs	1 bay leaf
1 whole garlic bulb	3 celery stalks, halved	1 tablespoon whole black peppercorns	8 cups water

To make the vegetable broth

1. In an electric pressure cooker, combine the garlic, onion, celery, carrots, collard greens, bay leaves, rosemary, parsley, ginger, and water.
2. Close and lock the lid and set the pressure valve to sealing. Select the Manual/Pressure Cook setting and cook for 20 minutes.
3. Once cooking is complete, allow the pressure to release naturally. Carefully remove the lid.
4. Using a large fine-mesh strainer, carefully strain the solids from the broth; discard the solids. Transfer the broth to an airtight container. Let cool completely.

CONTINUED

To make the chicken broth

1. In an electric pressure cooker, combine the chicken carcass, garlic, onion, celery, carrots, tomato, bay leaves, thyme, and water.
2. Close and lock the lid and set the pressure valve to sealing. Select the Manual/Pressure Cook setting and cook for 20 minutes.
3. Once cooking is complete, allow the pressure to release naturally. Carefully remove the lid.
4. Using a large fine-mesh strainer, carefully strain the solids from the broth; discard the solids. Transfer the broth to an airtight container. Let cool completely.

To make the seafood broth

1. In an electric pressure cooker, combine the shrimp shells, garlic, onion, celery, parsley, peppercorns, bay leaf, and water.
2. Close and lock the lid and set the pressure valve to sealing. Select the Manual/Pressure Cook setting and cook for 20 minutes.
3. Once cooking is complete, allow the pressure to release naturally. Carefully remove the lid.
4. Using a large fine-mesh strainer, carefully strain the solids from the broth; discard the solids. Transfer the broth to an airtight container. Let cool completely.

Storage Tip:

Broth can be stored in the refrigerator and used within 7 days or transferred to the freezer in a freezer-safe container for up to 3 months.

Variation:

For those with shellfish allergies, use a whole fish (including the bones) in place of the shrimp shells.

Vegetable Broth Per Serving (1 cup): Calories: 15; Total fat: 0 g; Saturated fat: 0g; Sodium: 0mg; Total carbohydrates: 3g; Sugar: 0g; Fiber: 0g; Net carbohydrates: 3g; Protein: 0g
Chicken Broth Per Serving (1 cup): Calories: 35; Total fat: 2g; Saturated fat: 0g; Sodium: 15mg; Total carbohydrates: 0g; Sugar: 0g; Fiber: 0g; Net carbohydrates: 0g; Protein: 5g
Seafood Broth Per Serving (1 cup): Calories: 21; Total fat: 1g; Saturated fat: 0g; Sodium: 32mg; Total carbohydrates: 0g; Sugar: 0g; Fiber: 0g; Net carbohydrates: 0g; Protein: 4g

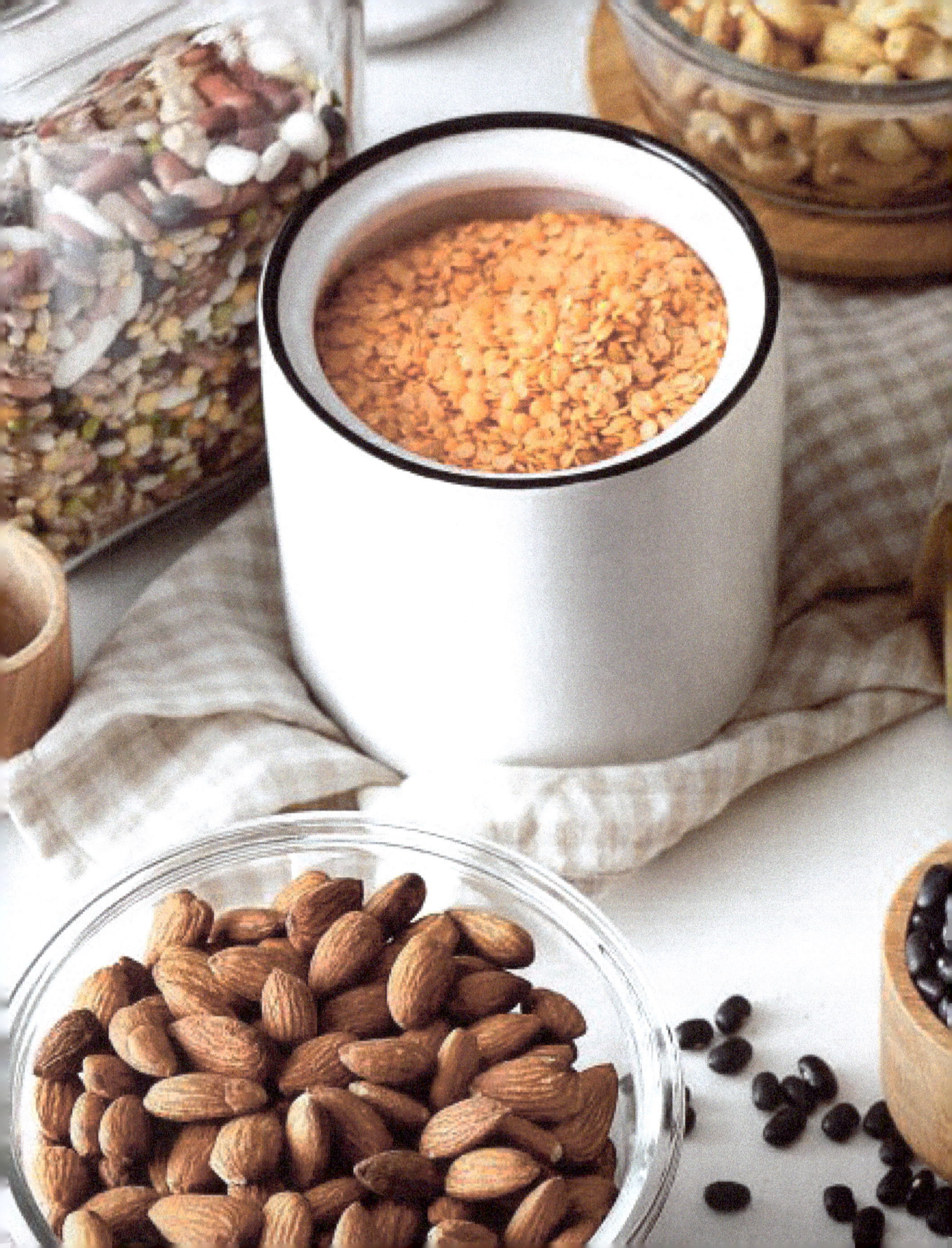

Measurement Conversions

	US STANDARD	US STANDARD (OUNCES)	METRIC (APPROXIMATE)
VOLUME EQUIVALENTS (LIQUID)	2 TABLESPOONS	1 FL. OZ.	30 ML
	¼ CUP	2 FL. OZ.	60 ML
	½ CUP	4 FL. OZ.	120 ML
	1 CUP	8 FL. OZ.	240 ML
	1½ CUPS	12 FL. OZ.	355 ML
	2 CUPS OR 1 PINT	16 FL. OZ.	475 ML
	4 CUPS OR 1 QUART	32 FL. OZ.	1 L
	1 GALLON	128 FL. OZ.	4 L
VOLUME EQUIVALENTS (DRY)	⅛ TEASPOON		0.5 ML
	¼ TEASPOON		1 ML
	½ TEASPOON		2 ML
	¾ TEASPOON		4 ML
	1 TEASPOON		5 ML
	1 TABLESPOON		15 ML
	¼ CUP		59 ML
	⅓ CUP		79 ML
	½ CUP		118 ML
	⅔ CUP		156 ML
	¾ CUP		177 ML
	1 CUP		235 ML
	2 CUPS OR 1 PINT		475 ML
	3 CUPS		700 ML
	4 CUPS OR 1 QUART		1 L
	½ GALLON		2 L
	1 GALLON		4 L

OVEN TEMPERATURES

FAHRENHEIT	CELSIUS (APPROXIMATE)
250°F	120°C
300°F	150°C
325°F	165°C
350°F	180°C
375°F	190°C
400°F	200°C
425°F	220°C
450°F	230°C

WEIGHT EQUIVALENTS

U.S. STANDARD	METRIC (APPROXIMATE)
½ OUNCE	15 G
1 OUNCE	30 G
2 OUNCES	60 G
4 OUNCES	115 G
8 OUNCES	225 G
12 OUNCES	340 G
16 OUNCES OR 1 POUND	455 G

References

Adams, O. Peter. (2013). "The impact of brief high-intensity exercise on blood glucose levels." *Diabetes, Metabolic Syndrome and Obesity: Targets and Therapy* 6: 113–122. doi:10.2147/DMSO.S29222.

American Diabetes Association. (n.d.). "Diagnosis." Diagnosis | ADA. Retrieved October 2, 2021, from Diabetes.org/a1c/diagnosis.

American Diabetes Association. (2020, February 1). "What is the diabetes plate method?" Diabetes Food Hub. Retrieved October 3, 2021, from DiabetesFoodHub.org/articles/what-is-the-diabetes-plate-method.html.

Carlson, O., B. Martin, K. S. Stote, et al. (2007). "Impact of reduced meal frequency without caloric restriction on glucose regulation in healthy, normal-weight middle-aged men and women." *Metabolism: Clinical and Experimental* 56(12): 1729–1734. doi.org/10.1016/j.metabol.2007.07.018.

Cefalu, W. T. (September 30, 2020). "Achieving type 2 diabetes remission through weight loss. National Institute of Diabetes and Digestive and Kidney Diseases." Retrieved October 4, 2021, from NIDDK.NIH.gov/health-information/professionals/diabetes-discoveries-practice/achieving-type-2-diabetes-remission-through-weight-loss.

Centers for Disease Control and Prevention. (June 15, 2021). "National Diabetes 2020 Statistics Report." Retrieved October 2, 2021, from CDC.gov/diabetes/data/index.html.

Centers for Disease Control and Prevention. (June 11, 2020). "Prediabetes—your chance to prevent type 2 diabetes." Retrieved October 5, 2021, from CDC.gov/diabetes/basics/prediabetes.html.

Colberg, Sheri R., Ronald J. Sigal, Jane E. Yardley et al. (November 2016). "Physical activity/exercise and diabetes: a position statement of the American Diabetes Association." *Diabetes Care* 39 (11): 2065–2079. doi.org/10.2337/dc16-1728.

Fuhrman J. (2018). "The hidden dangers of fast and processed food." *American Journal of Lifestyle Medicine* 12(5): 375–381. doi.org/10.1177/1559827618766483.

Gill, S., and S. Panda. (2015). "A smartphone app reveals erratic diurnal eating patterns in humans that can be modulated for health benefits." *Cell Metabolism* 22(5): 789–798. doi.org/10.1016/j.cmet.2015.09.005.

Gray, A., and R. J. Threlkeld. "Nutritional recommendations for individuals with diabetes." (Updated 2019 Oct 13). In: K. R. Feingold, B. Anawalt, A. Boyce et al., editors. South Dartmouth (MA): MDText.com, Inc.; 2000. NCBI.NLM.NIH.gov/books/NBK279012.

InformedHealth.org. Cologne, Germany: Institute for Quality and Efficiency in Health Care (IQWiG); 2006-. "Hyperglycemia and hypoglycemia in type 2 diabetes." [Updated 2020 Oct 22]. NCBI.NLM.NIH.gov/books/NBK279510.

Kwanbunjan, Karunee, Pornpimol Panprathip, et al. 2018. "Association of retinol binding protein 4 and transthyretin with triglyceride levels and insulin resistance in rural Thais with high type 2 dibetes risk." *BMC Endocrine Disorders* 18. BMCEndocrDisord .BioMedCentral.com/articles/10.1186/s12902-018-0254-2.

Luukkonen, P. K., S. Sädevirta, Y. Zhou, et al. (August 1, 2018). "Saturated fat is more metabolically harmful for the human liver than unsaturated fat or simple sugars." *Diabetes Care.* Retrieved November 14, 2021, from care.DiabetesJournals.org/content/41/8/1732.

Moro, T., G. Tinsley, A. Bianco, A., et al. (2016). "Effects of eight weeks of time-restricted feeding (16/8) on basal metabolism, maximal strength, body composition, inflammation, and cardio-vascular risk factors in resistance-trained males." *Journal of Translational Medicine* 14(1): 290. doi.org/10.1186/s12967-016-1044-0.

Poggiogalle, E., H. Jamshed, and C. M. Peterson. (2018). "Circadian regulation of glucose, lipid, and energy metabolism in humans." *Metabolism: Clinical and Experimental* 84: 11–27. doi.org/10.1016/j.metabol.2017.11.017.

Ravussin, E., R. A. Beyl, E. Poggiogalle et al. (August 2019). "Early time-restricted feeding reduces appetite and increases fat oxidation but does not affect energy expenditure in humans." *Obesity* 27(8): 1244–1254. 10.1002/oby.22518. PMID: 31339000; PMCID: PMC6658129.

Sapra, A., and P. Bhandari. "Diabetes Mellitus." (Updated September 18, 2021). StatPearls. NCBI.NLM.NIH.gov/books/NBK551501.

Stote, K. S., D. J. Baer, K. Spears et al. (2007). "A controlled trial of reduced meal frequency without caloric restriction in healthy, normal-weight, middle-aged adults." *American Journal of Clinical Nutrition* 85(4): 981–988. doi.org/10.1093/ajcn/85.4.981.

Sutton, Elizabeth, Robbie Beyl, Kate S. Early, et al. (2018). "Early time-restricted feeding improves insulin sensitivity, blood pressure, and oxidative stress even without weight loss in men with prediabetes." *Cell Metabolism* 27 (6): 1212–1221. doi.org/10.1016/j.cmet.2018.04.010.

Tinsley, G. M., J. S. Forsse, N. K. Butler et al. (2017). "Time-restricted feeding in young men per-forming resistance training: A randomized controlled trial." *Eur J Sport Sci.* 17(2): 200–207. doi: 10.1080/17461391.2016.1223173. Epub 2016 Aug 22. PMID: 27550719.

Index

THE COMPLETE TYPE 2 DIABETES COOKBOOK FOR BEGINNERS

Acknowledgments

I would like to thank my best friend and husband, Jace Warren. My husband and my three children continuously motivate me to live a long and healthy life with diabetes. I would like to thank my wonderful parents, Carol and Mark Barratt, along with my admirable in-laws, Kelly and Scott Warren. I would like to thank my darling grandma-in-law, Darlene Warren, who I have grown to view as my own grandma. She has type 2 diabetes and through this tough disease, we have found great joy while spending time together. I would like to thank my best friend, AnneMarie Rousseau, who also has diabetes and has dedicated her professional life as a healthcare professional. I would like to thank the editor, Georgia Freedman, and the Callisto team for all their hard work and dedication in creating this book. I appreciate all of you for your support, kindness, and profound impact.

About the Editor

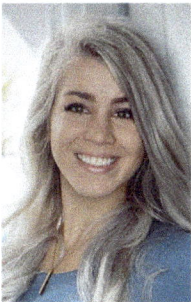

Ariel Warren is a Registered Dietitian Nutritionist (RDN) and a Certified Diabetes Care and Education Specialist (CDCES). She was diagnosed with type 1 diabetes at an early age, which has motivated her to dedicate her professional life to helping others with diabetes. Ariel graduated from Brigham Young University in Nutrition and Dietetics, then completed her dietetic internship at Utah State University. She then spent several years as a diabetes educator working at a local outpatient center. Today, Warren works as a healthcare provider through her online private practice and gives back as an author on diabetes, a speaker on optimizing control through tech and nutrition, and a creator of her online diabetes community.

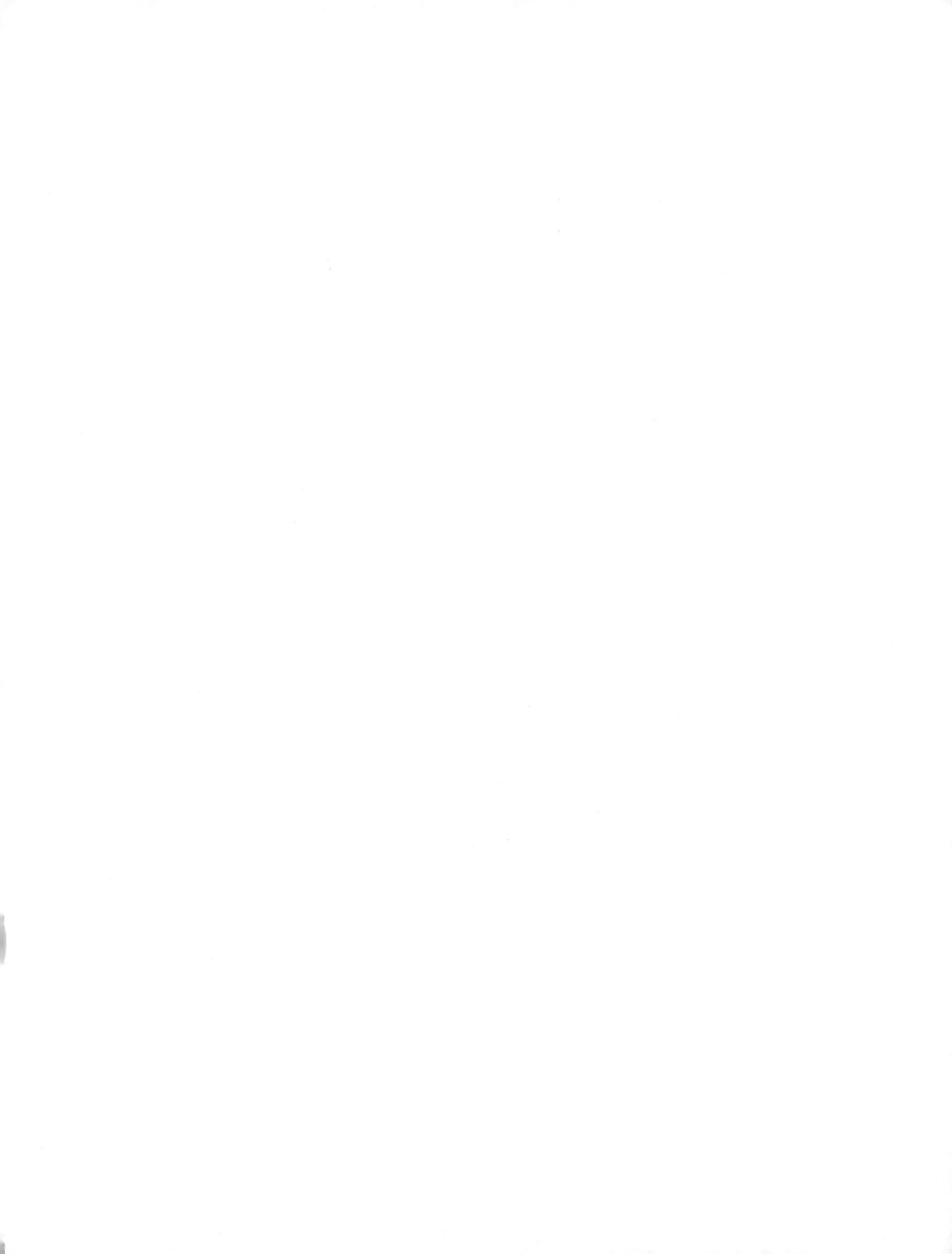

www.ingramcontent.com/pod-product-compliance
Lightning Source LLC
Chambersburg PA
CBHW061236270326
41930CB00022B/3484